Case Studies in Dementia

Volume 2

Case Studies in Dementia

Common and Uncommon Presentations

Volume 2

Edited by

Pedro Rosa-Neto
McGill University

Serge Gauthier
McGill University

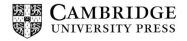

CAMBRIDGE
UNIVERSITY PRESS

University Printing House, Cambridge CB2 8BS, United Kingdom

One Liberty Plaza, 20th Floor, New York, NY 10006, USA

477 Williamstown Road, Port Melbourne, VIC 3207, Australia

314–321, 3rd Floor, Plot 3, Splendor Forum, Jasola District Centre,
New Delhi – 110025, India

79 Anson Road, #06–04/06, Singapore 079906

Cambridge University Press is part of the University of Cambridge.

It furthers the University's mission by disseminating knowledge in the
pursuit of education, learning, and research at the highest international
levels of excellence.

www.cambridge.org
Information on this title: www.cambridge.org/9781316638057
DOI: 10.1017/9781316941294

First edition © Cambridge University Press 2011
Second edition © Cambridge University Press 2021

First published 2011
Second edition 2021

Printed in Singapore by Markono Print Media Pte Ltd

A catalogue record for this publication is available from the British Library.

Library of Congress Cataloging-in-Publication Data
Names: Rosa-Neto, Pedro, editor. | Gauthier, Serge, 1950– editor.
Title: Case studies in dementia : common and uncommon presentations /
edited by Pedro Rosa-Neto and Serge Gauthier.
Description: Second edition. | Cambridge, United Kingdom ; New York, NY :
Cambridge University Press, 2020. | Includes bibliographical references and
index.
Identifiers: LCCN 2019035750 (print) | LCCN 2019035751 (ebook) |
ISBN 9781316638057 (paperback) | ISBN 9781316941294 (epub)
Subjects: MESH: Dementia–diagnosis | Diagnostic Techniques and
Procedures | Dementia–genetics | Biomarkers | Case Reports
Classification: LCC RC521 (print) | LCC RC521 (ebook) | NLM WM 220 |
DDC 616.8/31–dc23
LC record available at https://lccn.loc.gov/2019035750
LC ebook record available at https://lccn.loc.gov/2019035751

ISBN 978-1-316-63805-7 Paperback

Contents

Contents

Contributors

James T. Becker
Departments of Neurology, Psychiatry, and Psychology, University of Pittsburgh Alzheimer's Disease Research Center, Pittsburgh, PA, USA

Andrea L. Benedet
McGill University Research Centre for Studies in Aging, Douglas Research Centre, Integrated University Health and Social Services Centre; McGill University, Montreal, QC, Canada

Simona Maria Brambati, PhD
Centre Integrated University Health and Social Services Centre Sud; Research Center of the Montréal Geriatric Institute, Department of Psychology, Université de Montréal, QC, Canada

Aline Carvalho Campanha
Cognitive and Behavioral Neurology Research Group, School of Medicine, Federal University of Minas Gerais, Belo Horizonte, Brazil

Paulo Caramelli
Cognitive and Behavioral Neurology Research Group, School of Medicine, Federal University of Minas Gerais, Belo Horizonte, Brazil

Karoline Carvalho Carmona
Cognitive and Behavioral Neurology Research Group, School of Medicine, Federal University of Minas Gerais, Belo Horizonte, Brazil

Maria Teresa Carthery-Goulart
Center of Mathematics, Computing and Cognition (CMCC), Federal University of ABC, São Bernardo do Campo, São Paulo, Brazil

Mira Chamoun
McGill University Research Centre for Studies in Aging, Douglas Research Centre, Integrated University Health and Social Services Centre; McGill University, Montreal, QC, Canada

Laksanun Cheewakriengkrai
Phramongkutklao Hospital, Bangkok, Department of Neurology, Thailand

Parichita Choudhury
Department of Clinical Neurosciences, University of Calgary, Calgary, Alberta, Canada

Donnabelle Chu
Department of Clinical Neurosciences, University of British Columbia, BC, Canada

Renaud David
The Cognition Behavior Technology unit of the University Côte d'Azur, Nice University Hospital, and Claude Pompidou Institute, Nice, France

Fábio Henrique de Gobbi Porto
Department of Neurology, University of São Paulo, Brazil

Leonardo Cruz de Souza
Faculty of Medicine, Federal University of Minas Gerais, Belo Horizonte, Brazil

André Aguiar Souza Furtado de Toledo
Faculty of Medicine, Federal University of Minas Gerais, Belo Horizonte, Brazil

Eline Donders
Alzheimer Center and Department of Neurology, Neuroscience Campus Amsterdam, VU University Medical Center, Amsterdam, the Netherlands

Antoine Duquette
Movement Disorders Unit André Barbeau, Division of Neurology, Research Center of the Center Hospitalier de l'Université de Montréal, Montreal, QC, Canada

Christopher Feehan
Division of Neurology, University of British Columbia, Canada

Yuxue Feng
Department of Neurology, the Second Affiliated Hospital, Chongqing Medical University, Chongqing, China

Bruno F. A. L. Franchi
Royal Adelaide Hospital | RAH Department of Geriatric and Rehabilitation Medicine, Adelaide, Australia

Morris Freedman
Department of Medicine (Neurology), University of Toronto, Canada; Department of Medicine, Division of Neurology and Sam and Ida Ross Memory Clinic, Baycrest Health Sciences, Toronto, ON, Canada; Rotman Research Institute of Baycrest Centre, Canada

Calen Freeman
Department of Nursing, Baycrest Health Sciences, Toronto, ON, Canada, and Lawrence S. Bloomberg Faculty of Nursing, University of Toronto, ON, Canada

Leandro Boson Gambogi
Faculty of Medicine, Federal University of Minas Gerais, Belo Horizonte, Brazil

Serge Gauthier
McGill University Research Centre for Studies in Aging, Douglas Research Centre, Integrated University Health and Social Services Centre; McGill University, Montreal, QC, Canada

Cindy Giaume
The Cognition Behavior Technology unit of the University Côte d'Azur, Nice University Hospital, and Claude Pompidou Institute, Nice, France

Frédéric Potvin Gingras
André Barbeau Movement Disorders Unit, University of Montreal Hospital Center, Montreal, QC, Canada

Isabelle Gomez-Luporsi
The Cognition Behavior Technology unit of the University Côte d'Azur, Nice University Hospital, and Claude Pompidou Institute, Nice, France

Henrique Cerqueira Guimarães
Faculty of Medicine, Federal University of Minas Gerais, Belo Horizonte, Brazil

Marie Christine Guiot
The Neuro, Montreal Neurological Institute-Hospital, Montreal, Canada

Mindy Halper
Department of Nursing, Baycrest Health Sciences, Toronto, ON, Canada

Katharina Hein
Department of Neurology and Psychiatry, University Medical Centre, Georg-August University, Göttingen, Germany

Peter Hermann
German Center for Neurodegenerative Diseases (DZNE), Göttingen, Germany

Mirna Lie Hosogi
Department of Neurology, University of São Paulo, São Paulo (SP), Brazil

Philippe Huot
Movement Disorders Unit André Barbeau, Division of Neurology, Research Center of the Center Hospitalier de l'Université de Montréal, Montreal, QC, Canada

Masamichi Ikawa
Second Department of Internal Medicine (Neurology), Faculty of Medical Sciences, University of Fukui, Fukui, Japan; Department of Medical Genetics, University of Fukui Hospital, Fukui, Fukui Japan

Gordon Jewett
Department of Clinical Neurosciences, University of Calgary, Calgary, Alberta, Canada

Peter Johannsen
Danish Dementia Research Center, Department of Neurology, Rigshospitalet, Copenhagen University Hospital, Denmark

Nagaendran Kandiah
Department of Neurology, National Neuroscience Institute, Singapore

Ashan Khurram
Royal Adelaide Hospital | RAH Department of Geriatric and Rehabilitation Medicine, Adelaide, Australia

Julia Kofler
Department of Pathology, University of Pittsburgh Alzheimer's Disease Research Center, Pittsburgh, PA, USA

Lawrence Korngut
Department of Clinical Neurosciences, University of Calgary, Calgary, Alberta, Canada

Ian Law
Department of Clinical Physiology, Nuclear Medicine and PET, Rigshospitalet, Copenhagen University Hospital, Denmark

Elsa Leone
The Cognition Behavior Technology Unit of the University Côte d'Azur, Nice University Hospital, and Claude Pompidou Institute, Nice, France

Xiaofeng Li
Department of Neurology, the Second Affiliated Hospital, Chongqing Medical University, China

Yu Li
Department of Neurology, the Second Affiliated Hospital, Chongqing Medical University, China

Oscar L. Lopez
Departments of Neurology, Psychiatry, and Psychology, University of Pittsburgh Alzheimer's Disease Research Center, Pittsburgh, PA, USA

Thais Helena Machado
Department of Internal Medicine, Faculty of Medicine, Federal University of Minas Gerais, Belo Horizonte (MG), Brazil

Ian R. A. Mackenzie
Department of Pathology, University of British Columbia, Vancouver, BC, Canada

Sarinporn Manitsirikul
McGill University Research Centre for Studies in Aging, Douglas Research Centre, Integrated University Health and Social Services Centre; McGill University, Montreal, QC, Canada

Fadi Massoud
Department of Medicine, University of Montreal, Montreal, Canada

Akiko Matsunaga
Second Department of Internal Medicine (Neurology), Faculty of Medical Sciences, University of Fukui, Fukui, Japan

Sara Mohades
McGill University Research Centre for Studies in Aging, Douglas Research Centre, Integrated University Health and Social Services Centre; McGill University, Montreal, QC, Canada

Paige Moorhouse
Division of Geriatric Medicine, Department of Medicine, Dalhousie University & Nova Scotia Health Authority

Aurélie Mouton
The Cognition Behavior Technology unit of the University Côte d'Azur, Nice University Hospital, and Claude Pompidou Institute, Nice, France.

William S. Musser
Department of Neurology, University of Pittsburgh Alzheimer's Disease Research Center, Pittsburgh, PA, USA

Kok Pin Ng
Department of Neurology, National Neuroscience Institute, Singapore

Jørgen Erik Nielsen
Danish Dementia Research Center, Department of Neurology, Rigshospitalet, Copenhagen University Hospital, Denmark

Ricardo Nitrini
Department of Neurology, University of São Paulo School of Medicine, São Paulo (SP), Brazil

Leonard Numerow
Department of Radiology, University of Calgary, Calgary, Alberta, Canada

Michel Panisset
Movement Disorders Unit André Barbeau, Division of Neurology, Research Center of the University Hospital Centre, University of Montreal, Montreal, QC, Canada

Marlee Parsons
McGill University Research Centre for Studies in
Aging, Douglas Research Centre, Integrated
University Health and Social Services Centre; McGill
University, Montreal, QC, Canada

Tharick A. Pascoal
McGill University Research Centre for Studies in
Aging, Douglas Research Centre, Integrated
University Health and Social Services Centre; McGill
University, Montreal, QC, Canada

Gerald Pfeffer
Department of Clinical Neurosciences, University of
Calgary, Calgary, Alberta, Canada

Yolande Pijnenburg
Alzheimer Center and Department of Neurology,
Neuroscience Campus Amsterdam, VU University
Medical Center, Amsterdam, the Netherlands

Kely Quispialayasocualaya
McGill University Research Centre for Studies in
Aging, Douglas Research Centre, Integrated
University Health and Social Services Centre; McGill
University, Montreal, QC, Canada

Katrin Radenbach
Department of Neurology and Psychiatry, University
Medical Centre, Georg-August University, Göttingen,
Germany

Elisa de Paula França Resende
Cognitive and Behavioral Neurology Research Group,
School of Medicine, Federal University of Minas
Gerais, Belo Horizonte, Brazil

Philippe Robert
The Cognition Behavior Technology unit of the
University Côte d'Azur, Nice University Hospital, and
Claude Pompidou Institute, Nice, France

Ging-Yuek Robin Hsiung
Division of Neurology, Dept. of Medicine, University
of British Columbia, UBC Hospital, Vancouver BC,
Canada

Peter Roos
Danish Dementia Research Center, Department of
Neurology, Rigshospitalet, Copenhagen University
Hospital, Denmark

Pedro Rosa-Neto
McGill University Research Centre for Studies in
Aging, Douglas Research Centre, Integrated
University Health and Social Services Centre; McGill
University, Montreal, QC, Canada

Rodrigo A. Santibanez
Division of Neurology, Department of Medicine,
University of British Columbia, UBC Hospital,
Vancouver BC, Canada

Melissa Savard
McGill University Research Centre for Studies in
Aging, Douglas Research Centre, Integrated
University Health and Social Services Centre; McGill
University, Montreal, QC, Canada

Monica Shin
McGill University Research Centre for Studies in
Aging, Douglas Research Centre, Integrated
University Health and Social Services Centre; McGill
University, Montreal, QC, Canada

Bandit Sirilert
Phramongkutklao Hospital, Department of
Neurology, Bangkok, Thailand

Jean-Paul Soucy
PET centre, Brain Imaging Centre, Montreal
Neurological Institute, McGill University, Montreal,
QC, Canada

Jette Stokholm
Danish Dementia Research Center, Department of
Neurology, Rigshospitalet, Copenhagen University
Hospital, Denmark

Joseph Therriault
McGill University Research Centre for Studies in
Aging, Douglas Research Centre, Integrated
University Health and Social Services Centre; McGill
University, Montreal, QC, Canada

Marie-Pierre Thibodeau
Department of Medicine, University of Montreal,
Montreal, Canada

Linyan Tong
Department of Neurology, the Second Affiliated
Hospital, Chongqing Medical University, China

Paolo Vitali

McGill University Research Centre for Studies in Aging, Douglas Research Centre, Integrated University Health and Social Services CIUSSS du Centre et Nord-de-l'Île-de-Montréal; McGill University, Montreal, QC, Canada

M. Uri Wolf

Baycrest Health Sciences and Department of Psychiatry, University of Toronto, ON, Canada

Liyong Wu

Innovation Center for Neurological Disorders, Department of Neurology, Xuanwu Hospital, Capital Medical University, Beijing, China

Zongyi Xie

Department of Neurosurgery, the Second Affiliated Hospital, Chongqing Medical University, China

Makoto Yoneda

Department of Medical Genetics, Faculty of Nursing and Social Welfare Sciences, Biomedical Imaging Research Center, University of Fukui, Fukui, Japan

Inga Zerr

German Center for Neurodegenerative Diseases (DZNE), Göttingen, Germany

Preface

Typical dementia cases characterized by a slowly progressive amnestic syndrome in patients older than 65 years-old constitutes a highly prevalent condition in clinical practice. However, clinicians frequently encounter a significant number of atypical dementia cases featuring either rapid progression, or early onset (younger than 65 years old), or dominance of non-amnestic symptoms. As dementia constitutes a rapidly growing topic in neurology, case studies in dementia intends to illustrate advances in diagnosis of typical and atypical cases.

The first volume of Case Studies in Dementia focused on the classical presentations of typical and atypical dementias. Apart from typical Alzheimer's disease, we included cases of Alzheimer's disease associated with congophilic amyloid angiopathy, posterior cortical atrophy, behavioral presentation of Alzheimer's disease, and mixed pathology cases between Alzheimer's and vascular dementia. We also included various non-Alzheimer dementia cases.

On the spectrum of frontotemporal dementia, volume one describes presentations of the behavioral variant, semantic dementia, progressive non-fluent aphasia, and dementia with motor neuron disease. We also included a synucleinopathy case with Lewy body dementia and a poststroke and vascular dementia case following surgery with a Klüver–Bucy syndrome. There are cases of secondary dementias due to toxic encephalopathy and substance abuse. Regarding transmissible causes of dementia, volume one has chapters describing the clinical features of dementia cases secondary to neurosyphilis, HIV, Heidenhain variant of Creutzfeldt–Jakob, as well as Gerstmann–Sträussler–Scheinker disease. Finally, volume one closes with a section on dementias associated with genetic disorders. There are cases of adult-onset polyglucosan body disease, a disorder characterized by a deficiency of the glycogen-branching enzyme; another case of dementia due to genetic mitochondriopathy and Huntington's disease, which is a polyglutamine repeat disease.

This second volume highlights in its clinical cases the conceptual, genetic, and biomarker advances adopted by the recent operational definitions of dementing diseases. To this end, the first clinical case introduces the biomarker conceptual framework for investigating atypical dementia cases.

Subsequently, Chapter 2 provides insights regarding care planning in typical and atypical cases. On the spectrum of typical presentations, we included a asymptomatic and a typical case of Alzheimer's disease both diagnosed by second generation imaging agents. As atypical cases, we discuss an early-onset Alzheimer's disease and a case of cognitive decline associated with neurofibrillary tangle-predominant dementia. As for focal cortical syndromes, this volume includes cases of frontal variant due to Alzheimer's disease. There are cases of behavioral variant of frontotemporal degeneration due to C09orf75, MAPT17, progranulin, CHR3, and TARDBP mutations. The present volume also includes a case of posterior cortical atrophy and an intriguing case with the association between posterior cortical atrophy and logopenia. Regarding language presentations, there are cases of agrammatic, semantic, and logopenic presentations of primary progressive aphasia. There is also an interesting case illustrating alexia without agraphia associated with Pick's disease. A number of chapters illustrate dementia syndromes with motor manifestation such as progressive supranuclear palsy, Lewy body dementia, multiple system atrophy, normal pressure hydrocephalus as well as Wilson's and Parkinson's disease. We include two cases of dementia following cerebrovascular diseases. Regarding prion diseases, the reader will have the opportunity to contrast a Creutzfeldt–Jakob disease and fatal familial insomnia. We added a case of paraneoplastic syndrome and a case of Hashimoto's encephalopathy for illustrating autoimmune causes of dementia. The differential diagnosis of psychiatric conditions and dementia is exemplified in a case describing a patient with bipolar disorder. The second volume closes with an Appendix with the updated diagnostic criteria of the typical and atypical cases. We hope that this appendix would streamline the learning process for students and residents.

We would like to express our gratitude to the patients, their respective caregivers and family members who have contributed to this case book. We would like to thank the authors for their diligence, time, and patience to accomplish all tasks required and we would also like to thank Monica Shin, MSc, for her valuable voluntary assistance provided in this volume. On behalf of all authors, we would like to thank all our families, as well as the organizations for supporting our work in dementia research and clinical care.

We expect that the cases presented in this book would serve as an inspiration for the next generation of researchers and health professionals to advance the care of dementia patients.

A Young Missionary with Problems Quoting the Bible

Pedro Rosa-Neto, Monica Shin, Tharick A. Pascoal, Andrea L. Benedet,
Mira Chamoun, Jean-Paul Soucy, Kely Quispialayasocualaya,
and Serge Gauthier

1.1 Main Complaint

A 55-year-old priest who retired due to significant cognitive decline.

1.2 Clinical History

The patient came to the consultation accompanied by his wife who provided most of the history. She described her husband as a priest with persuasive and eloquent oratory, which was highly appreciated by their religious community. However, during the last 3 years, there was a clear impoverishment of the patient's ability to preach. During the services, he also started losing the thread of his narratives and getting confused on quoting the bible. His ability of multi-tasking in the church was impaired. A year later, he clearly acquired difficulties in retaining information regarding conversations as well as a hard time in organizing his day and accomplishing all the commitments of his agenda. Soon after, he started to forget contents of conversations and lost the ability to deal with calculations, and consequently, his financial affairs. He became unable to write. His wife also remarked the patient's inability to focus attention on his tasks. He also had a little insight regarding his present limitations.

Apart from a general reduction in motivation and social isolation, from the neuropsychiatric perspective, there was no history of disinhibition, reduced impulse control, substance-related disorders, stereotypical or ritualistic symptoms, hallucinations, or delusions. He was previously evaluated by a neurologist who diagnosed him with Alzheimer's disease (AD) based on clinical history, MRI, positron emission tomography (PET) using [^{18}F]fluorodeoxyglucose (FDG; Figure 1.1), and results of biomarkers from the cerebrospinal fluid (CSF). He was on 10 mg of donepezil every morning.

1.3 General History

This patient completed grade 12 and worked as a pastor and missionary until 53 years old. He was married once and had two daughters. He and his immediate family lived in many places with precarious urban infrastructure and sanitation including the sub-Saharan Africa. He was exposed to many tropical diseases, many of them not diagnosed. His previous medical history was negative for cardiovascular diseases, high blood pressure, hyperlipidemia, stroke, or diabetes. There was no history of current sleep disorders and cardiovascular, respiratory, urinary, sensory, or motor complaints.

1.4 Family History

His family history was negative for early-onset familial AD (EOFAD) but positive for late-onset familial AD (LOFAD; grandmother) and amyotrophic lateral sclerosis (ALS; father).

1.5 Examination

The physical examination was unremarkable. During the mental status exam, he was cooperative, attentive, and responsive and partially oriented in time and space. The immediate recall was normal. He was not able to correctly tell the months in reverse order. He made few mistakes on the serial 7. The design copy and clock drawing were abnormal. Reading and repetition were normal. He was capable of writing a simple sentence, but his writing skills were impaired. The single word and the sentence comprehension were normal. The content of language was impoverished. Verbal and semantic fluency was reduced. Anterograde memory evoked by a delayed recall showed deficits that were not corrected by cueing. The capacity for abstraction was abnormal. Montreal Cognitive Assessment (MoCA) was 12/30 (visuospatial: –4, serial 7: –3, fluency: –1, abstraction: –2, delay recall: –5, orientation: –3) and the Mini-Mental State Examination (MMSE) was 17/30 (orientation: –3, serial 7: –5, delay recall: –3, design copy: –1). The patient was not capable of executing motor sequences. No significant perseveration, omission, or commissions were observed. The rest of the neurological examination was normal.

1.6 Diagnostic Workup

This patient had normal hematology, biochemistry, and autoimmune profile. He had an EEG without features of Creutzfeldt–Jakob disease. An MRI ruled out brain infarcts or white matter hyperintensities (Fazekas = 0) with a mild progression of hippocampal atrophy (Scheltens = 2–3). MRI diffusion imaging was normal. The FDG PET scan showed reduction on the FDG uptake in the precuneus, temporoparietal cortex, sparing the posterior cingulate. The CSF analysis showed $A\beta1$–42 of 397 pg/mL, a total tau (t-tau) of 488 pg/mL, a hyperphosphorylated tau (p-tau) of 61 pg/mL, and an ATI index of 0.52. The patient engaged in a research protocol and also had a positive amyloid PET and tau PET showing high uptake in the temporal lobe (mesial, basal, and neocortical), precuneus, inferior parietal cortex, orbitofrontal cortex, and amygdala (Braak stage 5; see Figure 1.1). He had a genetic assessment that was negative for MAP, C09orf72, progranuline, PS1, PS2, and APP mutations. He was an APOE 2/3 carrier.

1.7 Diagnosis

The diagnostic in this case is sporadic young-onset AD with evidence of the AD pathophysiological processes.

1.8 Discussion

The objective of this case report is to highlight the use of appropriated criteria for AD biomarkers in clinical practice. In the present case, our patient had the clinical history of a dementing disease characterized by an insidious onset, a clear-cut history of worsening of cognition and cognitive presentation encompassing language, memory, and executive deficits in the absence of cardinal features or other neurodegenerative conditions. The term "young-onset dementia" designates symptom onset before 65 years of age. The cutoff of 65 years is arbitrary and reflects aspects related to retirement age rather than any biological criteria.

As the prevalence of non-AD pathologies is higher in young-onset dementia, the knowledge of AD pathophysiology might affect the clinical management, in terms of therapeutics with cholinesterase inhibitors. Biomarkers are useful for providing to the caregiver and family members information regarding disease prognosis. In case of a positive family history, the presence of AD pathophysiology could guide genetic investigation.

The same logic is applicable to atypical dementia cases, which are clinically characterized by the predominance of behavioral, visuospatial, or language symptoms instead of the typical amnestic presentation of AD. As in young-onset cases, there is a higher

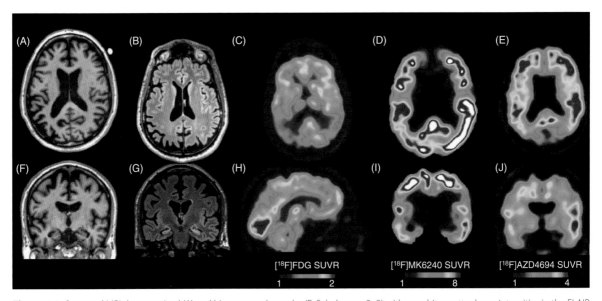

Figure 1.1 Structural MRI shows parietal (A) and hippocampal atrophy (F; Scheltens = 2–3) with no white matter hyperintensities in the FLAIR imaging (B, G; Fazekas = 0). FDG PET shows bilateral hypometabolism in the precuneous (H) and temporoparietal cortex (C; L ≫ R). Tau PET (D, I) shows deposition in limbic, temporal, and frontal cortices, sparing primary motor cortex (Braak stage 5). Amyloid PET (E, J) showed high load in the precuneous, posterior cingulate, inferior parietal, and frontal cortices.

Table 1.1 Biomarkers available in clinical practice

		Amyloid load	Tau load	Neuronal injury	Vascular pathology	Dopamine depletion
Fluid	CSF	Aβ1–42	p-tau181	t-tau	Plasma CSF albumin ratio	
	Blood	Not clinically useful (NCU)	NCU	NCU		
Imaging	MRI	NCU	NCU		FLAIR T2*	
	PET	[18F]Amyvid [18F]NeuraCeq [18F]Vizamyl	None	[18F]FDG		
	SPECT			99mTc hexamethylpropyleneamine oxime [HMPAO] 99mTc-ethylene cysteine [ECD]		DAT scans

Table 1.2 Summary of appropriated use criteria of biomarkers in clinical practice

	MRI	CSF	FDG	Amyloid imaging
Late-onset dementia	Yes	No	No	No
Typical MCI or prodromal AD	Yes	No	No	No
Young-onset dementia	Yes	Yes	Yes	Yes
Atypical features	Yes	Yes	Yes	Yes

(i.e., blood, saliva, or CSF) or imaging biomarkers (MRI and PET). Biomarkers can be also classified according to their respective pathophysiological processes, for example, biomarkers of amyloid pathology, tau pathology, and neurodegeneration (Table 1.1).

Although guidelines for dementia management suggest that at primary level, a computer tomography would be sufficient for ruling out structural abnormalities in patients with cognitive decline, MRI has better sensitivity to detect tumors, vascular abnormalities, or brain atrophy commonly observed in dementia populations. Structural MRI allow for assessing the ventriculomegaly in patients with clinical symptoms of normal pressure hydrocephalus. T2 fluid-attenuated inverse recovery (FLAIR) allows for assessing white matter hyperintensities associated with microvascular changes as well as the pulvinar sign in Creutzfeldt–Jakob disease. Frequently, the white matter hyperintensities are reported as Fazekas scores or similar metrics. T2* gradient echo images permit the identification of hemosiderin deposits associated with microbleeds. MRI-restricted diffusion sequences are capable of detecting abnormalities associated with Creutzfeldt–Jakob disease. Assessment of structural abnormalities has been frequently utilized in dementia. In fact, reduction of hippocampal volume assessed with MRI has been considered as an important biomarker of neuronal damage in AD for a long time and can be quantified by visual inspection of appropriated acquisitions. The Scheltens score for medial temporal atrophy as well as similar scales has been frequently used to this end.

prevalence of other pathological substrates rather than AD among patients with atypical dementias.

Although the knowledge of disease processes underlying atypical cases has modest but significant clinical applications, this scenario might change dramatically with the introduction of preventive pharmacological therapies since the identification of the specific neuropathological processes is a sine qua non condition for disease-modifying therapies. Despite significant progresses of biomarker research, there is a limited number of clinically useful biomarkers, which are summarized in Table 1.1. The most acceptable indications for biomarkers in dementia are summarized in Table 1.2.

Biomarkers indicative of cerebrovascular disease or the presence of AD pathophysiology are the most accepted in clinical practice. Regarding their origin, biomarkers can be classified into fluid biomarkers

Fluid biomarkers have the advantage of simultaneously quantifying many pathophysiological aspects associated with dementias. They are easily obtained, and the cost is lower than imaging biomarkers. The major drawback concerns high variability across methods and laboratories. Only Aβ1–42, p-tau, and t-tau have clinical relevance for quantifying brain amyloidosis, tau phosphorylated at threonine 181, and total tau protein, respectively. Possibly, neurofilament light chain will become a clinically useful biomarker in the CSF and plasma.

The Aβ peptide, composed of 42 amino acids (Aβ1–42), is the result of the cleavage of transmembrane amyloid precursor protein by the sequential proteolytic action of beta and gamma secretases. The resultant Aβ1–42 is highly hydrophobic and lipophilic and therefore continuously aggregates as Aβ plaques in the extracellular brain compartment. As such, its concentration in the CSF declines as a function of plaque formation in the brain. Changes in CSF concentrations of Aβ are considered as one of the earliest pathophysiological events in AD, occurring more than 10 years before the dementia onset.

The microtubule-associated protein, tau, is abundantly present within neurons and glia compartment, where they play a role in cytoskeleton stabilization. In AD, neurofibrillary tangles occur as a result of hyperphosphorylation of tau proteins. Current research supports the concept that tau and phosphorylated tau are also released into the extracellular space, resulting in increased CSF tau concentrations in AD. It has been postulated that early forms of hyperphosphorylated tau and Aβ aggregates (oligomers) are the most neurotoxic forms of amyloid and tau; however, the mechanisms by which amyloid and tau leads to neurodegeneration remains elusive.

PET constitutes a powerful technique to identify and quantify metabolic abnormalities and deposits of amyloid and tau aggregates in the brain of patients with AD. Fluorodeoxyglucose ([^{18}F]FDG) is the most diffused PET imaging technique to investigate dementias particularly to differentiate AD from frontotemporal dementias. FDG is currently conceptualized as a marker of neuronal injury. The FDG signature in AD is characterized by hypometabolism in the hippocampus, posterior cingulate, precuneous, inferior parietal, lateral temporal, and mid-prefrontal cortices.

PET amyloid imaging agents such as [^{18}F]-Amyvid, [^{18}F]NeuraCeq, and [^{18}F]Vizamyl have been approved in various countries for clinical use; however, the price and the availability of PET cameras constitute a limitation for their uses. Although the recent introduction of tau imaging agents brings new perspectives to the research in disease pathophysiology and therapeutics, tau imaging agents are not yet indicated for clinical practice. It is possible that these agents could be used to differentiate patients with neurofibrillary tangle predominant dementia from frontotemporal dementia. Presently, "The Imaging Dementia – Evidence for Amyloid Scanning (IDEAS)" study will provide definitive answers regarding the clinical utility of amyloid imaging agents in clinical practice.

Single photon emission computed tomography (SPECT) remains an imaging modality more accessible than PET to investigate patients with atypical dementia. 99mTc hexamethylpropyleneamine oxime (HMPAO) and 99mTc-ethylene cysteine (ECD) have been clinically utilized; however, their contributions on the differential diagnosis of dementia remain debatable. The SPECT DaTscans (Ioflupane I 123 injections, also known as phenyltropane) is a radiopharmaceutical agent that shows depletion of dopaminergic projections to the basal ganglia. Although DaTscan is FDA approved to investigate cases of atypical Parkinson's disease, only few studies systematically assessed its value in the postmortem diagnosis of Lewy body dementia.

In the case presented here, the use of biomarkers provided sufficient evidence corroborating the diagnosis of AD. This information supported the indication of cholinesterase inhibitor and provided to the family relevant information necessary to take decisions regarding the care of this patient at home. The presence of AD pathophysiology also played a role on the decision to investigate genetic factors in this patient.

Specifically, in this case, there was a convergence between the CSF and imaging biomarkers toward the presence of AD pathophysiology. However, borderline or conflicting biomarker results are frequently observed in clinical practice. The choice between fluid and imaging biomarkers depends on the availability of the methodology (PET imaging agents) or clinical circumstances such as the use of anticoagulation (contraindication for lumbar puncture) or pacemaker (contraindication for MRI). A clinical equivalence between imaging and CSF amyloid biomarkers has been shown. In fact, information regarding fluid and imaging biomarkers were described in this case report because the patient was a participant in a research protocol.

It is important to emphasize that a positive biomarker in the context of patients with atypical dementia should be carefully interpreted considering that frequent comorbidity between pathophysiological processes have been extensively described in various cohorts. Although biomarkers of amyloid and tau pathologies certainly advanced our understanding regarding pathophysiology of dementia, their clinical uses remain limited. These biomarkers will play a crucial role in the context of future interventions targeting specific disease process such as tau and amyloid.

1.9 Take-Home Messages

1. Biomarkers have a modest but significant impact on the management of patients with young-onset or atypical dementia.
2. There is a limited number of biomarkers that are considered useful in clinical practice.
3. Biomarkers play an important role on clinical trials for AD by excluding individuals without AD pathophysiology.

Further Reading

Atri A. Imaging of neurodegenerative cognitive and behavioral disorders: practical considerations for dementia clinical practice, 1 ed: Elsevier B.V., 2016.

Dubois B, Feldnam HH, Jacova C, et al. Advancing research diagnostic criteria for Alzheimer's disease: the IWG-2 criteria. *Lancet Neurol.* 2014;13:614–629.

Gauthier S, Patterson C, Chertkow H, et al. 4th Canadian Consensus Conference on the Diagnosis and Treatment of Dementia. *Can J Neurol Sci.* 2012;39:S1–S8.

Jack Jr CR, Albert MS, Knopman DS, et al. Introduction to the recommendations from the National Institute on Aging-Alzheimer's Association workgroups on diagnostic guidelines for Alzheimer's disease. *Alzheimers Dement.* 2011;7:257–262.

McKhann GM, Knopman DS, Chertkow H, et al. The diagnosis of dementia due to Alzheimer's disease: recommendations from the National Institute on Aging-Alzheimer's Association workgroups on diagnostic guidelines for Alzheimer & Dementia disease. *Alzheimers Dement.* 2011;7:263–269.

Niemantsverdriet E, Valckx S, Bjerke M, Engelborghs S. Alzheimer's disease CSF biomarkers: clinical indications and rational use. *Acta Neurol Belg* 2017;117:591–602.

Risacher S, Saykin A. Neuroimaging biomarkers of neurodegenerative diseases and dementia. *Semin Neurol.* 2013;33:386–416.

Care Planning and Decision-Making through the Stages of Dementia

Paige Moorehouse

2.1 Clinical History

A 72-year-old male is accompanied by his wife to his ambulatory memory clinic appointment. He has recently been assessed by a vascular surgeon in relation to his 5.8 cm abdominal aortic aneurysm (AAA). The surgeon has planned an open repair of the aneurysm, and refers the patient to the preoperative clinic for assessment. As part of the standard preoperative clinic assessment process, the patient undergoes a frailty screen using the Frailty Assessment for Care Planning Tool (FACT),[1] which utilizes caregiver input and objective cognitive testing (three-word recall, clock-drawing task) to assess frailty across four key domains: mobility, social situation, function, and cognition (Figure 2.1). The patient's frailty level is determined to be severe, largely driven by his cognitive and functional impairments. While there are no perioperative concerns, his nurse assessor has concerns about the patient's frailty and cognitive status, in particular, whether he truly understands the risks and benefits of the proposed surgery; therefore, she makes an urgent referral to the memory clinic, 1 week in advance of the scheduled aneurysm repair.

In the memory clinic, a more detailed cognitive history was taken to understand the trajectory and nature of the cognitive and functional deficits noted on the FACT screen. While the patient did not self-identify any memory concerns, at the memory clinic, his wife described a gradual decline in his cognition and function over the last several years. She indicated that 4 years ago he began falling behind on bill payments and occasionally forgot to take his antihypertensive medication, so she took over these tasks. Two years ago, when his driver's license expired, she "convinced" him not to renew it, her concerns stemming from three occasions where he'd gotten lost in familiar areas when driving alone and several driving infractions she'd witnessed as his passenger. Over the last 18 months, she has taken on all of the cooking and cleaning, and in the last 8 months, has regularly needed to remind him to bathe and put on clean clothing. Sometimes he requires hands-on help to manage the mechanics of dressing. She does not have any formal homecare assistance but has disengaged from many of her own social activities due to his agitation when she is out of the home for more than an hour.

There is no history of perceptual disturbance, depression, or neurovegetative symptoms. He reads the newspaper daily, although he usually cannot recall what he has read. He enjoys visits from his grandchildren, although he infrequently refers to them by name. He has had no behavioral issues or significant personality change, although she notes him to be more irritable with the grandchildren and more reliant on a fixed daily routine. There has been no change in his gait, balance, or physical strength.

Of his upcoming surgery, the patient's wife says, "I'm worried about what it will mean for him, but if this is what he wants to do, I'll support him in whatever way I can."

2.2 General History

Other than the AAA, the patient has no chronic health conditions. He has a remote history of smoking (25 pack years, quit 20 years ago) and does not consume alcohol. He achieved a grade 12 education and worked in trades as a plumber.

2.3 Family History

There is no family history of dementing illness.

2.4 Examination

General examination reveals a gentleman who is pleasant and cooperative. There are no lateralizing neurologic deficits, but there is bilateral paratonia notable in the upper extremities. His gait and balance are intact.

Consistent with the objective cognitive testing score from the FACT screen, testing with the Mini-Mental State Examination (MMSE)[2] reveals a score of 18/30, losing points for orientation to date, day, month, year, name of hospital, floor, 0/3 word recall, 2/5 spelling "world" backward, and incorrect intersecting pentagon diagram copying. Testing with the Frontal Assessment Battery (FAB)[3] reveals a score of 6/18 losing points in all domains (abstraction, verbal fluency, praxis, conflicting instructions, inhibitory control) except environmental autonomy. He is aware that he has "a problem with [my] blood supply," but is unable to provide any detail around the proposed surgery nor the outcomes associated with continued surveillance.

2.5 Special Studies

A CT of the head completed 2 months earlier when he sustained a fall revealed small vessel ischemic disease and mild cerebral atrophy in keeping with his age.

2.6 Diagnosis

Moderate stage mixed vascular/Alzheimer's-type dementia. The patient does not have capacity for decision making regarding management of his AAA.

2.7 Discussion

This patient's case exemplifies some of the common challenges to dementia care in modern day medicine.[4] First, the well-documented challenge of dementia recognition in clinical practice is compounded when patients with dementia have other competing health issues for which standard of care therapies such as surgery, chemotherapy, renal replacement therapy, and so on might be recommended. Non-memory clinics often overlook the impact of a dementia diagnosis on capacity or outcomes, and rely on self-report measures for much of their patient history. Second, in the absence of objective cognitive assessment, many cases of dementia among older adults are overlooked despite frequent medical visits. Many patients are able mask considerable cognitive impairment during brief physician encounters, and the gestalt clinical suspicion approach for memory clinic referrals often fails to detect the subtle and varied nature of cognitive deficits in dementia. The routine evaluation of frailty using tools that also objectively test cognition can help prevent this common, but troubling, oversight.

Like adulthood, frailty is a life stage through which every older adult will pass; it is in fact the result of optimal medical care. Frailty is the vulnerability to poor health outcomes that occurs as a result of accumulation of health deficits over the life course. Dementia is a common and important driver of frailty to the degree that dementia stage as described in standard rating scales such as the Functional Assessment Staging Tool (FAST)[5] positively correlates with frailty stage: moderate dementia indicates (at least) moderate frailty. The recent proliferation of

studies examining the importance of frailty in predicting outcomes with standard of care interventions provides a new lens through which to underscore the importance of early and routine detection of dementia. Not only does a diagnosis of dementia stand to influence treatment decisions for the dementia itself, it should also inform treatment decisions for other chronic comorbidities outside of the memory clinic. Establishing decision-making capacity and appointing a substitute decision maker when required should be key considerations for any clinical setting that serves an aging patient population before carrying out standard of care therapies. Appropriate care planning and delivery for dementia patients is contingent on early detection and diagnosis followed by careful consideration of frailty level and goals of care to achieve the best possible outcomes for this vulnerable population.

The FACT (Figure 2.1) was developed by two geriatricians as a standardized method for assigning a Clinical Frailty Scale[6] score for nonexperts in geriatrics. The FACT assesses frailty across the domains of cognition, mobility, function, and social situation, using a combination of caregiver reports and objective measures to achieve a proper understanding of the patient's baseline and degree of deficits. To assess cognition, the assessor uses items from the Mini-Cog (i.e., the ability to recall three unrelated items following the clock-drawing test)[7] and the memory axes of the Brief Cognitive Rating Scale[8] (i.e., the ability to recall current events, the current US president, and the names of first-degree relatives). Mobility, function, and social vulnerability scores are assigned then verified according to a collateral historian (usually a caregiver) due to challenges with self-report of function when cognitive impairment is prevalent. Final frailty level is interpreted as the worst score in any of the four domains (i.e., severe cognition infers severe frailty level). The FACT currently has applications in a variety of clinical settings, including cardiovascular surgery, anesthesia preoperative clinics, outpatient nephrology, and in medical oncology; areas in which the utility of a standardized frailty measurement for making informed healthcare decisions can directly affect patient outcomes.

2.8 Case Outcome

In this patient's case, routine frailty screening followed by a diagnosis of dementia and disclosure

FACT FINAL SCORING SHEET

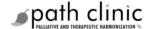

path clinic
PALLIATIVE AND THERAPEUTIC HARMONIZATION

MOBILITY IS AT BASELINE? ☑ YES O NO			COGNITION IS AT BASELINE? O YES O NO
Baseline Mobility	**Social**	**Function**	**Cognition**
1. Thriving	O Fit, exercises regularly (among fittest for age)	O In charge of organizing social events	O Still working at job or high level hobby	O **Thriving**: Impresses others with memory and thinking
2 & 3. Normal Aging	O Active/exercises occasionally	O Socializes weekly & would have a caregiver if needed	O Subjective impairment (i.e. does everything on own but finds things more difficult)	O **Normal**: Family (caregiver) is not concerned about memory O **Normal**: Collateral unavailable
4. Vulnerable	☑ Starting to slow down and often tired during the day	O Socializes less than weekly OR might not have a caregiver if needed	O Not dependent on others but symptoms often limit activities	O **Vulnerable**: Minor deficits on testing (**Cognitive impairment, not dementia**) O **Vulnerable**: Family (caregiver) concerned but normal testing
5. Mild	O Walking slower and regularly uses (or should use) a cane or walker	O Socializes rarely	O Needs help with some instrumental activities of daily living (IADLS) (e.g. housework, banking or medications)	O **Mild stage dementia**: Vague/incorrect recall of current events, can recall name of US president
6. Moderate	O Needs help of another person when using stairs, walking on uneven ground, or getting in/out of bath O Has fallen more than once in the past 6 months, excluding slip on ice	☑ Mostly house-bound	O Needs assistance or dependent for IADLS and cueing with basic activities of daily living (BADLS) (e.g. help choosing what to wear or requires reminders to bathe)	O **Moderate stage dementia**: Incorrect recall of US President, can recall name of children/spouse O No collateral present
7. Severe	O Always needs someone's help when walking OR unable to propel self in manual wheelchair	O House-bound and isolated OR caregiver stress/or no available caregiver to meet care needs	☑ Needs hands on help with BADLS (bathing, toileting, dressing)	☑ **Severe stage dementia**: Unable to name children, spouse or siblings
8. Very Severe	O Bed bound, unable to participate in transfers	O Unable to participate in any social exchange, even when visited	O Dependent for all aspects of daily life	O **Very severe stage dementia**: Limited language skills with few words verbalized

Compatible with: Rockwood K. CMAJ. 2005;173:489-495; Borson S. Int J Geriatr Psychiatry. 2000;15:1021-1027; Reisberg B. Psychopharmacol Bull. 1988;24:629-636.

FINAL FRAILTY LEVEL __SEVERE__   Signature __M Lawrence__   Date __SEPTEMBER 29, 2017__

Figure 2.1 FACT utilizes caregiver input and objective cognitive testing (three word recall, clock drawing task) for assessing frailty across four key domains: mobility, social situation, function, and cognition.

of dementia stage became the anchor for communication with his wife (also his identified substitute decision maker). First, the diagnosis of dementia and the associated assessment of the patient's understanding and appreciation of the risks and benefits of the proposed surgery made it clear that deferring to the patient's stated preference would not be following an informed directive. Identifying the substitute decision maker, in this case, his wife was the next step in decision-making. His wife admitted that she had concerns about her husband's ability to engage with the conversation they had with his surgeon, but felt uncomfortable raising her concerns in the absence of a cognitive diagnosis.

Next, the concept that successful standard of care treatment (in this case open repair of his AAA) was intended to prolong survival was introduced. In this case, in the absence of other comorbidities, successful treatment of the AAA would mean survival and progression from the moderate to the severe stage of dementia. The functional correlates of severe stage

dementia (i.e., needing hands-on help with bathing and dressing) were described and discussed with the decision maker. A subsequent discussion sought to determine how the patient's premorbid values fit with the current plan of pursuing life-prolonging measures in the face of moderate stage dementia. The patient's wife indicated that her interpretation of his preference would be to avoid interventions that would increase the likelihood of surviving to progress to severe or very severe stage dementia. She also expressed relief at the notion of forgoing the proposed procedure and having more time "with him as he is now." Further discussion centered around decision-making for future unrelated health crises using a structured process.[9]

After completion of the cognitive assessment and discussion, the surgery was canceled. The patient continued to live at home with his wife in relatively stable health. He was admitted to hospital 9 months later with acute coronary syndrome (ACS) for which he received palliative management and died in hospital.

2.9 Take-Home Message

People with dementia are, by virtue of their impairment, frail and additionally often have several other comorbidities, relying heavily on the healthcare system as a consequence. In the absence of routine screening for frailty and cognitive impairment, many frail and cognitively impaired patients move through the specialized healthcare system unrecognized.[10] This may contribute to poor health outcomes as a result of inappropriate self-directed care decisions or unsuitable applications of standard of care therapies for non-dementia comorbidities. Beyond honing the art of dementia treatment and diagnosis, the clinician has a responsibility to advocate for those patients who might otherwise not have their cognitive deficits detected and thereby miss out on the opportunities and benefits of appropriate decision-making that follow.

References

1. Clark DA, Khan U, Kiberd BA, et al. Frailty in end-stage renal disease comparing patient, caregiver, and clinician perspectives. *BMC Nephrol.* 2017;18(148):1–8.

2. Folstein MF, Folstein SE, McHugh PR. "Mini-mental state." A practical method for grading the cognitive state of patients for the clinician. *J Psychiatr Res.* 1975;12(3):189–198.

3. Dubois B, Slachevsky A, Litvan I, Pillon B. The FAB: a Frontal Assessment Battery at bedside. *Neurology.* 2000;55 (11):1621–1626.

4. Moorhouse P. Care planning in dementia: tips for clinicians. *Neurodegener Dis Manag.* 2014;4 (1):57–66.

5. Reisberg B. Functional assessment staging (FAST). *Psychopharmacol Bull.* 1988;24(4):653–659.

6. Rockwood K, Song X, MacKnight C, et al. A global clinical measure of fitness in elderly people. *CMAJ.* 2005;173(5):489–495.

7. Borson S, Scanlan J, Brush M, Vitaliano P, Dokmak A. The mini-cog: a cognitive "vital signs" measure for dementia screening in multi-lingual elderly. *Int J Geriatr Psychiatry.* 2000;15 (11):1021–1027.

8. Reisberg B, Ferris SH. Brief Cognitive Rating Scale (BCRS). *Psychopharmacol Bull.* 1988;24 (4):629–636.

9. Moorhouse P, Mallery LH. Palliative and therapeutic harmonization: a model for appropriate decision making in frail older adults. *J Am Geriatr Soc.* 2012;60: 2326–2332.

10. Bradford A, Kunik ME, Schulz P, Williams SP, Singh H. Missed and delayed diagnosis of dementia in primary care: prevalence and contributing factors. *Alzheimer Dis Assoc Disord.* 2009;23 (4):306–314.

A Young Man with Memory and Walking Difficulties

Monica Shin, Mira Chamoun, Tharick A. Pascoal, Melissa Savard, Jean-Paul Soucy, Marie Christine Guiot, Pedro Rosa-Neto, and Serge Gauthier

3.1 Main Complaint

A young 41-year-old man with memory problems and walking difficulties.

3.2 Clinical History

A young man came for a consultation accompanied by his father. He reported that his problems started at the age of 30 when he noticed fatigue and incapacity to accomplish his tasks at work. He was having difficulties remembering names of his colleagues and committed numerous mistakes as a clerk. When relocated to perform easier tasks at the store, he struggled to follow instructions. The cognitive deficits progressed to the point that he had to quit his job. As he was not able to manage his financial affairs anymore, his father became his caregiver since his wife abandoned him terrified by his progressive cognitive decline. His Montreal Cognitive Assessment (MoCA) declined by 6 points in 4 years. At age 34 years, he experienced difficulties in walking and started using a walker to avoid falls.

3.3 General History

He had thalassemia minor, with no clinical impact. He also used illicit drugs such as ecstasy and marijuana.

3.4 Examination

The physical examination conducted 10 years after the first manifestation of Alzheimer's disease (AD) was unremarkable. During the mental status exam, he was cooperative, attentive, and responsive, although showing some degree of time and space disorientation. His immediate recall was impaired. He was not capable of spelling backward. He made mistakes on the serial 7s. The figure copy and clock drawing were abnormal. Anterograde memory evoked by a delayed recall showed deficits, which were partially corrected by cueing. His speech was mildly slurred. The verbal fluency was reduced. He scored 20 on the MMSE and 14 on the MoCA.

During the neurological exam, the cranial nerves were normal. The motor exam revealed normal and symmetric strength. The tonus was symmetrically increased. He had hyperreflexia of all four limbs, bilateral plantar response, sustained clonus of both ankles, and showed decreased bilateral hand and foot tapping. Primitive reflexes (glabellar, palmomental, and snout reflexes) were present. Sensory examination was unremarkable. Cerebellar examination was within the limits of normality. His gait was spastic with a narrow base.

3.5 Family History

His mother died in 1981, at the age of 43, as a consequence of Gerstmann-Sträussler-Scheinker disease (GSS). Her brain necropsy revealed congophilic angiopathy, diffuse cortical neuronal loss, neuritic plaques, and status spongiosis of the neuropil, Kuru plaques in the parieto-occipital cortex and the cerebellum. The cholinergic innervation was reduced in the medial frontal cortex.[1] Recent reassessment of the pathological material with current pathology techniques ruled out the presence of the prion protein (PRNP) but revealed cotton wool amyloid formations on the tissue. To the best of their knowledge, there was no other individual affected by a neurodegenerative or psychiatric condition in their family.

3.6 Laboratorial Assessment

Blood tests showed that the plasma ceruloplasmin level was at 272 mg/L (220–480). The screen for HIV-1 and HIV-2 were both negative. A genetic study was negative for PRNP. The neuropsychological testing revealed a significant decline in all spheres of cognition. [^{18}F]fluorodeoxyglucose (FDG) positron emission tomography (PET) images showed a marked (~30%; Figure 3.1c and d) deterioration of uptake in multiple cortical areas, including the temporal lobes (both lateral and the hippocampal formations), the parietal lobes and, to a lesser extent, the frontal lobes. The amyloid imaging showed increased accumulation

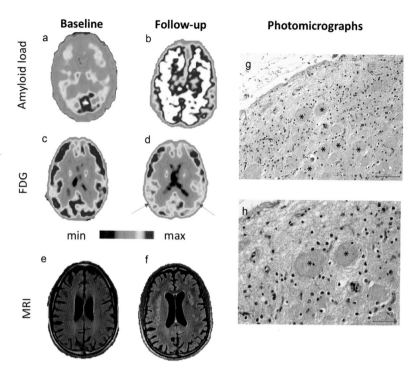

Baseline   **Follow-up**   **Photomicrographs**

Amyloid load

a   b

FDG

c   d

min ▬▬ max

MRI

e   f

g

h

Figure 3.1 Representative images of a baseline assessment of amyloid load (a, b) with PET [^{11}C]PIB, [^{18}F]FDG (c, d), MRI FLAIR images (e, f), and photomicrographs obtained from paraffin sections of formaldehyde-fixed brain tissue stained with hematoxylin-eosin (HE) at 10× (g) and 20× (h). Note the fast rate of increase of PIB load in a 24-month follow-up, the decline in cortical metabolism (blue arrows), ventricular dilation (f; red arrow), and cortical atrophy (f). HE stains reveals round, eosinophilic CWP (*) displacing normal structures in the cortical areas at 10× and 20×.

of the tracer with a cortical pattern, involving at a low level the frontal, temporal, and parietal cortices, with a much higher uptake in the occipital regions (~45%; Figure 3.1a and b). There was also significant increased uptake in the striatum, thalamus, brain stem, and cerebellum. Fluid-attenuated inversion recovery magnetic resonance imaging (FLAIR MRI) of brain without enhancement showed diffuse cerebral volume loss, including the cerebellum and no signs of white matter or cerebrovascular disease (Figure 3.1e and f). A repeat amyloid imaging conducted 24 months later showed significant uptake of tracer in various brain regions including the striatum. CSF revealed $AB_{1-42} = 338.25$ pg/mL, T-tau = 926.75 and p-tau = 139.3.

3.7 Follow-Up

Subsequent genetic analysis revealed no mutations for the amyloid precursor protein (APP) and the presenilin 2 (PSEN2) genes, but it was positive for presenilin 1 (PSEN1) mutation (c.1250G>C, p. Gly417Ala). Cholinesterase inhibitors were recommended, and the patient progressed from cognitive and motor impairments. He was admitted in a long-term care facility and developed spastic tetraparesis and mutism.

3.8 Diagnosis

This patient has Alzheimer's disease (AD) with dementia according to the NIA-AA research framework criteria,[2] or Alzheimer's disease with spastic paresis associated with a PS1 mutation (c.1250G>C, p.Gly417Ala).

3.9 Discussion

This case illustrates a young-onset (<65 years old) cognitive syndrome associated with motor symptoms in an individual with family history positive for GSS in a first-degree relative.

GSS is caused by mutations in the prion protein (PRNP) gene and might show autosomal dominant pattern in familial cases. GSS cases are characterized by young-onset dementia, motor manifestations including limb weakness, progressive limb and truncal ataxia, dysarthria, and cognitive decline. In GSS patients, PET-FDG shows reduced cerebellar metabolism and amyloid-PET study is typically negative. The absence of PRNP mutations, cortical hypometabolism, and the retention of amyloid in the PET scans refuted the GSS diagnosis and motivated the reanalysis of the anatomopathological diagnosis of his mother. In fact, the anatomopathological diagnosis of

GSS was conducted in 1981, which predates the first descriptions of prions or the genetic forms of AD as well their respective mutations. In addition, the identification of cotton wool amyloid plaques (CWP; also described after 1981), and the absence of immunoreactivity for PRNP in the anatomopathological specimens further motivated the investigation of the three genes causative of autosomal dominant AD.[3,4]

Autosomal dominant AD (ADAD) is associated with genetic mutations in the APP, PS1, and PS2 genes. ADAD is associated with young-onset dementia frequently accompanied by atypical features. These mutations enhance the amyloidogenic degradation of the APP and the generation of high tissue concentrations of toxic species of amyloid. PS1 protein constitutes part of the gamma secretase complex involved in the cleavage of APP into Aβ species.[5-7] The PS1 (p. Gly417Ala) mutation revealed by the sequencing analysis is new. Although no specific functional analysis was performed yet, the fact that this mutation has been recently reported in a Korean Family supports its pathogenicity.

Although spastic paraparesis in AD was described by Barrett in 1913, the definitive association between spastic paraparesis with a PSEN1 mutation was introduced only in 1997.[8] It has been reported significant phenotypes for PS1 mutations associated with spastic paraparesis. For example, while the spastic paraparesis in our case emerged as a dominant phenotype, the PS1 (p.Gly417Ala) case described in Korea had early-onset AD with Parkinsonism. Furthermore, a wide range of phonotypical expressions exist even within a single family.[3]

The age at disease onset was estimated during the third decade for both cases. The disease onset was characterized by a clear progressive amnestic and dysexecutive syndrome. However, during the course of the disease, while our patient developed a motor phenotype characterized by spastic paraparesis, the Korean case developed a Parkinsonian phenotype. Although pathological phenotypes remain unavailable for both cases, the findings reported in our patient's mother's necropsy supports the progressive paraparesis with cotton wool plaque phenotype. Indeed, there is a higher incidence of cerebral amyloid angiopathy and rates of amyloid deposition and spasticity in carriers of mutations located in the second half (>200 codon) of the PS1 gene.[2] It is important to emphasize that dementia either precedes or follows spastic paresis in PS1 mutations. The mechanism underlying these phenotypic variations remain unclear.[9,10] Autosomal dominant spastic paresis without dementia has been found in mutations on the spastin gene (SPG4), atlastin gene (SPG3A), nonimprinted gene in Prader-Willi syndrome/angelman gene (SPG6), and kinesin family member gene (SPG10).[11-14]

Cotton wool plaques variant was first described by Crook and colleagues in 1998.[4] Although cotton wool plaques constitute an important pathological feature of PS1 spastic paraparesis in AD, it has also been described in sporadic late-onset AD. Contrasting with mature amyloid plaques, cotton wool plaques are larger (5×), eosinophilic, and invisible to Congo red stain. The link between cotton wool plaques and motor degeneration remains elusive.

3.10 Take-Home Messages

1. PS1 mutation constitutes a plausible differential diagnosis in patients with dementia with motor symptoms.
2. Given the wide range of phenotypes, biomarkers of AD pathophysiology provide useful guidance in the diagnostic workup of patients with cognitive impairment and motor symptoms.
3. Be aware about phenotypic variances within family carriers of PS1 mutation.

References

1. Robitaille Y, Wood PL, Etienne P, et al. Reduced cortical choline acetyltransferase activity in Gerstmann-Sträussler syndrome. *Prog Neuropsychopharmacol Biol Psychiatry*. 1982;6(4–6):529–531.

2. Jack CR Jr, Bennett DA, Blennow K, et al. NIA-AA Research Framework: toward a biological definition of Alzheimer's disease. *Alzheimers Dement*. 2018;14 (4):535–562. doi: 10.1016/j. jalz.2018.02.018.

3. Mann DM, Pickering-Brown SM, Takeuchi A, Iwatsubo T; Members of the Familial Alzheimer's Disease Pathology Study Group. Amyloid angiopathy and variability in amyloid beta deposition is determined by mutation position in presenilin-1-linked Alzheimer's disease. *Am J Pathol*. 2001;158 (6):2165–2175.

4. Goate A, Chartier-Harlin MC, Mullan M, et al. Segregation of a missense mutation in the amyloid precursor protein gene with familial Alzheimer's

disease. *Nature.* 1991;349 (6311):704–706.

5. Levy E, Carman MD, Fernandez-Madrid IJ, et al. Mutation of the Alzheimer's disease amyloid gene in hereditary cerebral hemorrhage, Dutch type. *Science.* 1990;248(4959):1124–1126.

6. Smith MJ, Kwok JB, McLean CA, et al. Variable phenotype of Alzheimer's disease with spastic paraparesis. *Ann Neurol.* 2001; 49(1):125–129.

7. Mehta ND, Refolo LM, Eckman C, et al. Increased Abeta42(43) from cell lines expressing presenilin 1 mutations. *Ann Neurol.* 1998; 43(2):256–258.

8. Crook R, Verkkoniemi A, Perez-Tur J, et al. A variant of Alzheimer's disease with spastic paraparesis and unusual plaques due to deletion of exon 9 of presenilin 1. *Nat Med.* 1998;4 (4):452–455.

9. Scheuner D, Eckman C, Jensen M, et al. Secreted amyloid beta-protein similar to that in the senile plaques of Alzheimer's disease is increased in vivo by the presenilin 1 and 2 and APP mutations linked to familial Alzheimer's disease. *Nat Med.* 1996;2(8):864–870.

10. Hsiao K, Baker HF, Crow TJ, et al. Linkage of a prion protein missense variant to Gerstmann-Sträussler syndrome. *Nature.* 1989;338(6213):342–345.

11. Reid E, Dearlove AM, Rhodes M, Rubinsztein DC. A new locus for autosomal dominant "pure" hereditary spastic paraplegia mapping to chromosome 12q13, and evidence for further genetic heterogeneity. *Am J Hum Genet.* 1999;65(3):757–763.

12. Reed JA, Wilkinson PA, Patel H, et al. A novel NIPA1 mutation associated with a pure form of autosomal dominant hereditary spastic paraplegia. *Neurogenetics.* 2005;6(2):79–84.

13. Zhao X, Alvarado D, Rainier S, et al. Mutations in a newly identified GTPase gene cause autosomal dominant hereditary spastic paraplegia. *Nature Genet.* 2001;29:326–331.

14. Durr A, Davoine C-S, Paternotte C, et al. Phenotype of autosomal dominant spastic paraplegia linked to chromosome 2. *Brain.* 1996;119:1487–1496.

Elderly Man Repeating Questions about Upcoming Appointments

Serge Gauthier, Mira Chamoun, Tharick A. Pascoal, Jean-Paul Soucy, and Pedro Rosa-Neto

4.1 Case History

A 75-year-old, right-handed man accompanied by his wife presented at initial consultation, with a history of mild difficulties with short-term recall for the past 2 years. Although he wrote down the time and place of upcoming appointments accurately, he repeatedly sought reassurance from his wife about them. He kept rechecking where things had been deposited. There was some hesitation for words during conversations.

He had no difficulties playing bridge, paying his bills, driving his car, helping with grocery shopping, and putting dishes away at the proper location. He was independent for self-care.

He was sad because one of his sons was going through a recent divorce and he had been put on citalopram 2 months prior to the initial visit.

4.2 Past Medical History

He was in good general health, taking low doses of a statin and of an antihypertensive drug. He had uneventful cataract surgery.

4.3 Family History

Although his mother did not have dementia, some of his maternal aunts and uncles were reported to have had Alzheimer's disease (AD) in their 80s.

4.4 Social History

The patient was born in Montreal and completed a university degree in accounting. He worked in business management until he retired at age 65. He lives in his condo with his wife, and they have two sons and three grandchildren.

4.5 Initial Clinical Examination

The patient was fully cooperative during the examination. His blood pressure was 120/80, pulse 60 and regular. His general neurologic examination was normal for his age.

Cognitive assessment was performed in his mother tongue, English. His Mini-Mental State Examination (MMSE) score was 23/30, with errors in orientation to time (2) and place (1), impaired recall (3), and impaired drawing (1). His (MoCA) version 7.1 score was 18/30, with errors in visuospatial/executive tasks (3), animal naming (1), delayed recall (5), and orientation (3).

4.6 Clinical Diagnosis

The patient was initially diagnosed with mild dementia probably due to AD. Donepezil was prescribed at 5 mg a day.

4.7 Additional Clinical Investigations

A head computed tomography (CT) scan without infusion done 3 days after the initial consultation showed mild frontoparietal and cerebellar atrophy with mildly prominent ventricles. No significant cerebrovascular disease identified.

A positron emission tomography (PET)-glucose scan performed 1 month after the initial consultation showed hypometabolism of the posterior cingulum as well as both mesiotemporal regions (Figure 4.1).

4.8 Clinical Course

The patient was seen after 6 months of treatment with donepezil 5 mg a day, which was well tolerated despite slight nose dribbling (rhinorrhea) and a pulse of 48/min. The MMSE score improved to 25, although the family did not see an improvement, finding him repeating the same thing, and at times being unsure of himself, whereas at other times being very sharp. The donepezil dose was not increased because of concern about the asymptomatic bradycardia.

After 18 months of treatment with donepezil 5 mg a day, there had been no clinical change in the patient's daily routine, the pulse was 60, and the MMSE score was back to 23.

After 22 months of treatment with donepezil 5 mg the patient needed to be accompanied and helped with directions when driving his car, the pulse was 48, and the MMSE score was 22. Because of the inability to increase the donepezil to 10 mg, the patient and family chose a switch to the transdermal

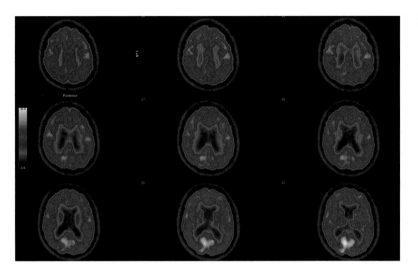

Figure 4.1 PET-glucose.

rivastigmine patch. Unfortunately, a skin reaction to the patch despite topical steroids caused a switch back to donepezil 5 mg a day.

After 3 years of treatment with donepezil and 5 years into his illness, the patient was stable in his daily routine, the MMSE score was 25. He expressed interest in participating in a research study.

4.9 Additional Research Investigations

A research 3T brain MRI was performed, showing diffuse brain atrophy with predominant atrophy in the inferior parietal, posterior cingulate, and precuneus cortices bilaterally and symmetrically. Hippocampus had bilateral atrophy, particularly on the left side (Figure 4.2a).

An amyloid PET scan using [18F] NAV4694 showed amyloid positivity with a pattern of deposition expected in patients with AD, predominantly in the posterior cingulum, precuneus, lateral temporal, and mesioprefrontal cortices (Figure 4.2b).

A tau PET scan using [18F] MK6240 showed tau deposition in the mesiobasal (transentorhinal, entorhinal, hippocampus, fusiform gyrus) and lateral temporal cortices, predominantly on the right side. These were none to very low [18F]MK6240 binding in the posterior cingulate, precuneus, and lateral temporal cortices (Figure 4.2c).

4.10 Discussion

This case of typical AD illustrates many useful clinical and research findings.

A clinical diagnosis of probable AD is facilitated by the availability of a reliable patient and informant, the latter being essential for a true assessment of decline in activities of daily living, changing mood, and emerging behaviors. Anosognosia has been found even in MCI subjects, correlates with AD-type biomarkers, and is a predictor of progression.[1] Furthermore, a reliable history combined with basic neurological assessments has been useful for many years toward the clinical diagnosis of "probable AD."[2]

Mood changes are common in early AD and should be treated prior to use of cholinesterase inhibitors (CIs). Scales such as the Minimal Behavioral Impairment (MBI-C) are useful to bring out subtle neuropsychiatric symptoms in MCI or early dementia stages of AD.[1]

CIs can be well tolerated despite age and bradycardia.[3] Their use requires periodic monitoring (every 6 months) when there is initiation, dose change, or switch to an alternative CI.

Patients with probable AD can be clinically stable for years using currently available drugs, a stable environment, and control of vascular risk factors. This stability has been more evident in current years and is a partial reason why randomized clinical trials (RCT) comparing putative disease-modifying drugs to placebo added on to regular care are not successful: there is clinical stability in most patients on placebo over 18 months.[4] This should not discourage patient's participation in RCT, but we need to improve our trials, designs, and outcomes.

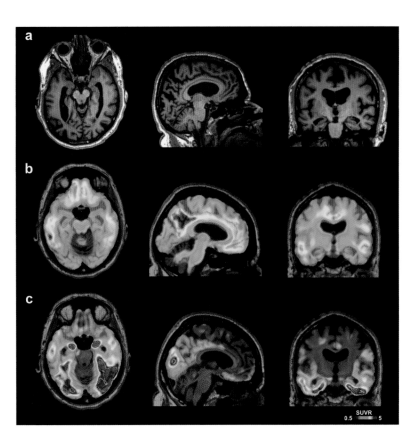

Figure 4.2 (a) MRI, (b) amyloid PET, (c) tau PET.

The utility of biomarkers in typical late-onset AD is debatable. An anatomic scan such as CT or MRI of the brain is generally done in memory clinics, but not felt to be required in routine clinical practice according to the Canadian Consensus Conference on Dementia unless there are specific clinical indications such as early onset, asymmetry on neurologic examination, and risk factors for stroke.[5]

The need for a PET-glucose scan could be argued on similar arguments and a consensus meeting has concluded that for a patient with a diagnosis of dementia who has undergone the recommended baseline clinical and structural brain imaging evaluation and who has been evaluated by a dementia specialist, but whose underlying pathological process is still unclear, preventing adequate clinical management, a [18F]-fluorodeoxyglucose (FDG)-PET scan should be obtained for differential diagnosis purposes.[6] It may have to be repeated after a minimum time of 12 months in atypical or unclear dementia syndromes.[7]

Similar arguments are being put forward for use of amyloid PET imaging. The original amyloid ligand PiB[8] using 11C is available in some research centers with ready access to a cyclotron, whereas the 18F ligands are more readily available commercially, and their clinical utility has been assessed by consensus meetings.[9]

The sensitivity and selectivity of tau PET scans in AD are being studied and are currently limited to research protocols.[10,11]

One other option for many countries and clinical sites is the use of lumbar puncture with measurements of ß42 and tau protein levels. Many international groups are looking at the clinical utility of these CSF biomarkers for clinical practice and hoping that blood markers will be proven useful.[12]

4.11 Summary

This patient with clinically probable AD can be well managed with family support and current medications. He and his family were interested in participation in research and other such patients should be encouraged to do so. The research can be observational or therapeutic.

There are different types of imaging tests available depending on the typical or atypical presentation or progression of the disease, as illustrated in other cases throughout this book.

References

1. Therriault J, Ng KP, Pascoal TA, et al. Anosognosia predicts propagation of default mode network metabolic deficits and clinical progression to dementia. *Neurology*. 2018;90(11):e932–e939.

2. McKhann GM, Knopman DS, Chertkow H, et al. The diagnosis of dementia due to Alzheimer's disease: recommendations from the National Institute on Aging-Alzheimer's Association workgroups on diagnostic guidelines for Alzheimer's disease. *Alzheimer Dement*. 2011;7:263–269.

3. Ismail Z, Agüera-Ortiz L, Brodaty H, et al. The Mild Behavioral Impairment Checklist (MBI-C): a rating scale for neuropsychiatric symptoms in pre-dementia populations. *J Alzheimers Dis*. 2017;56:929–938.

4. Drugs for cognitive loss and dementia. *Med Lett Drugs Ther*. 2017;59:155–161.

5. Gauthier S, Albert M, Fox N, et al. Why has therapy development for dementia failed in the last two decades? *Alzheimers Dement*. 2016;12:60–64.

6. Soucy JP, Bartha R, Bocti C, et al. Clinical applications of neuroimaging in patients with Alzheimer's disease: a review from the 4th Canadian Consensus Conference on the Diagnosis and Treatment of Dementia 2012. *Alzheimer Res Ther*. 2013;5 (Suppl. 1):S3.

7. Bergeron D, Beauregard JM, Guimond J, et al. Clinical impact of a second FDG-PET in atypical/ unclear dementia syndromes. *J Alzheimers Dis*. 2016;49 (3):695–705.

8. Klunk WE, Engler H, Nordberg A, et al. Imaging brain amyloid in Alzheimer's disease with Pittsburgh Compound-B. *Ann Neurol*. 2004;55:306–319.

9. Laforce R, Rosa-Neto P, Soucy JP, et al. Canadian Consensus guidelines on use of amyloid imaging in Canada: update and future directions from the Specialized Task Force on Amyloid Imaging in Canada (STAG). *Can J Neurol Sci*. 2016;43:503–512.

10. Marquié M, Normandin MD, Vanderburg CR, et al. Validating novel tau positron emission tomography tracer [F-18]-AV-1451 (T807) on postmortem brain tissue. *Ann Neurol*. 2015;78:787–800.

11. Maass A, Landau S, Baker SL, et al. Comparison of multiple tau-PET measures as biomarkers in aging and Alzheimer's disease. *NeuroImage*. 2017;157:448–463.

12. Olsson B, Lautner R, Andreasson U, et al. CSF and blood biomarkers for the diagnosis of Alzheimer's disease: a systematic review and meta-analysis. *Lancet Neurol*. 2016;15:673–684.

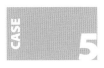
A Devoted Wife with an Atypical Finding

Tharick A. Pascoal, Monica Shin, Mira Chamoun, Serge Gauthier, and Pedro Rosa-Neto

5.1 Case History

Mrs. M is a 79-year-old active and independent lady who lives with her 88-year-old husband. She has been serving as his caregiver since his AD dementia diagnosis. Both cohabit with each other in the same house for more than 30 years. She has been responsible for maintaining their home, preparing meals, and has taken care of their financial affairs for many years. Mrs. M was invited to participate in a 3-year longitudinal study, as a cognitively healthy person, involving magnetic resonance imaging (MRI) and positron emission tomography (PET) scans for amyloid plaques, neurofibrillary tangles, and glucose metabolism.

5.2 Medical History

Mrs. M is a right-handed, 160 cm tall lady who weighs approximately 60 kg with a BMI of 23.4. She has been diagnosed with hypertension 4 years ago, without suffering from diabetes or hyperlipidemia. She was never hospitalized or has experienced head injuries. She was never a smoker and consumed approximately half a serving of alcohol per week during most of her life.

5.3 Family History

There is no relevant family history.

5.4 General History

Mrs. M was raised in Montreal since she was 4 years old after her family emigrated from Poland in order to escape from World War II. She obtained a bachelor's degree in general sciences in 1957 at McGill University and continued her postgraduate studies at the State University of Iowa, where she graduated with a master's degree in speech pathology in 1959. Right after, she was hired by the Montreal Children's Hospital as a speech pathologist where she worked for 4 years until she got pregnant. Since then, she dedicated the rest of her life to take care of her family. As a housewife, she strived to prepare natural and balanced meals and to encourage routine exercise to her husband and children.

5.5 Clinical and Cognitive Assessments

During her participation in the imaging study, Mrs. M was extensively assessed, clinically and cognitively. In the baseline and follow-up visits, Mrs. M showed intact clinical and cognitive evaluations. In the follow-up examination, her clinical dementia rating (CDR) sum of boxes score was 0, indicating no symptoms of dementia; there was no impairment in her memory, orientation (with time, person, and place), judgments and problem solving, community affairs, home and hobbies, and personal care. Her scores for Mini-Mental State Examination (MMSE) and Mild Behavioural Impairment Checklist (MBI-C) were 30/30 and 0/3 on all questions, respectively. Two tests from Delis–Kaplan Executive Function System (D-KEFS) were administered: (1) Trail Making Test to assess flexibility of thinking on a visual-motor sequencing task and (2) Semantic Verbal Fluency Test to measure letter fluency, category fluency, and category switching. In the Trail Making Test, Mrs. M completed Part A in 46 s without errors and Part B in 180 s with one sequence and two switching errors. In the Semantic Verbal Fluency Test, she named 16 animals and 14 boys' names correctly without any set loss or repetition errors in 60 s each. Finally, she scored 12/25 on immediate and 10/25 on delayed recall in the Logical Memory 1A Test. According to her Geriatric Depression Scale score of 1/30, Mrs. M was not depressed, and she reported that she does not notice worsening of her memory and that there is no concern regarding her memory or thinking. Overall, her cognitive health was in excellent condition with absence of any psychiatric symptoms. In addition, there was absence of abnormal cognitive performances or behaviors that appeared to be impulsive or obsessive. Mrs. M did not report any changes in her sleep and appetite or any impairment in her usual activities.

5.6 MRI and PET Acquisitions

Mrs. M underwent four different scanning procedures: (1) structural MRI, (2) [18F]fluorodeoxyglucose

(FDG) PET for glucose metabolism, (3) [¹⁸F]NAV4694 PET for amyloid plaques, and (4) [¹⁸F]MK6240 PET for neurofibrillary tangles. The MRI scan showed diffuse atrophy with hippocampal atrophy bilaterally. MRI FAIR imaging showed no infarctions and mild white matter hyperintensities load. The [¹⁸F]FDG scan showed mild to moderate reduction of glucose uptake in the posterior portion of the cingulate and precuneus cortices. Amyloid and tau PET scans showed accumulation in an AD pattern with deposition predominantly in the posterior cingulate, precuneus, lateral temporal, and inferior parietal cortices (Figure 5.1).

5.7 Diagnosis

The individual is a cognitively normal elderly with a research diagnosis of preclinical AD stage 2 since she performed normally in the cognitive assessments and had a positive amyloid scan with structural and metabolic abnormalities typically found in AD. Three years later, by the occasion of the clinical follow-up of the study, she had an additional tau PET scan that revealed typical deposition of Braak stage V with neurofibrillary tangles in the superior temporal but not in the primary visual cortex. Despite the presence of significant AD pathophysiology in Mrs. M's brain, she remained without experiencing any cognitive difficulties in the 3-year follow-up.

5.8 Discussion

This case describes a cognitively intact woman carrier of abnormal brain amyloid and neurofibrillary tangles deposition, as well as neurodegenerative abnormalities detected by in vivo neuroimaging techniques. This case illustrates a notion that has gained interest since the beginning of the 1990s: the concept of "reserve." Specifically, here, reserve is discussed in the context of a patient cognitively stable for 3 years with preclinical AD stage 2 and advanced tau pathology (Braak stage V).

The idea that "reserve" explains the disassociation between the degree of brain pathology and the clinical manifestation of AD has significantly evolved since it was proposed by Katzman and colleagues, who used this concept for conciliating the presence of normal cognition in individuals with postmortem evidence of brain AD pathology. Although researchers have significantly increased our understanding of "reserve" since then, little is known regarding the coexistence of brain abnormalities measured with in vivo biomarkers for amyloid, tau, and neurodegeneration with cognitive deficits and progression to dementia. Therefore, there has been a growing interest in cases such as Mrs. M, where there is a disconnection between the in vivo biomarkers' result and the progression to dementia over time. In this regard, it is postulated that there is a combination of different types of

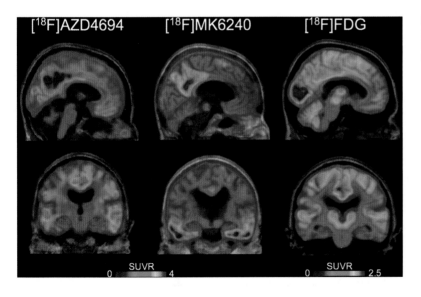

Figure 5.1 PET scans overlaid in the patient's structural MRI showed abnormalities compatible with a diagnosis of Alzheimer's disease.

reserves that stand in the way between pathology and disease progression.

The reserve could be passive, also known as *brain reserve*, which is the innate capability of the brain to sustain its function against brain damage. This type of reserve is postulated as *passive* since it refers to the amount of pathology that the brain can tolerate until the damage reaches a certain threshold and the clinical manifestation be established. The degree of brain reserve, thus the vulnerability to dementia, varies depending on the individual. Importantly, brain reserve is determined by existing quantitative elements such as brain size, number of synapses, and the abundance of neuronal networks and not by the brain's reactive processes toward injury. Factors that influence brain reserve include, but are not limited to, innate intelligence (IQ) and genetic components.

On the other hand, a reserve could be *active*, where the brain attempts to counteract the damages by using preexisting cognitive strategies or new compensatory methods. Under this construction, individuals with the same brain size could have different cognitive outcomes with the same amount of brain harm. This form of compensate is postulated to have two subtypes. One form of active reserve is called *neural compensation*, where the brain uses alternative structures or networks, shifting operations to circuits not normally used in response to brain damage. Importantly, compensation is not considered as part of the usual brain feedback and therefore involves the recruitment of structures or networks not engaged in the typical brain functioning. The other form is called *cognitive reserve*, which can be interpreted as the "software" of the brain; this involves cognitive paradigms that manage to endure and sustain the brain function through a more efficient use of the brain networks normally involved in the response to increased task demands. Therefore, cognitive reserve is present in both healthy and impaired individuals. Major factors that determine cognitive reserve include intellectual elements such as the level of education and occupational attainment, as well as lifestyle elements such as social/physical activities and hobbies. For example, linguistic ability at childhood was found to be one of the constituents of cognitive reserve. Furthermore, individuals that possess high intellectual ability, education, and socioeconomic status were found to be more likely to develop an engaged lifestyle, which in turn contributes to the maintenance of verbal intelligence, buffering against cognitive decline.

Among the factors already postulated to increase brain or cognitive reserve, Mrs. M has an education level above the average of a normal elderly population. Mrs. M formerly enjoyed exercise, walking almost every day with her husband around the city, and often she challenged herself with steeper walking routes to stay healthy. When it comes to her diet, Mrs. M does not restrict herself, always consuming the food that she craves. She is not vegetarian or vegan and always incorporates meats into her diet. Mrs. M does not have a significant intake of sweets or snacks and does not consume soft drinks, even since she was a child. In addition, Mrs. M likes to read, mostly nonfiction novels about traveling and current events around the world, she enjoys playing games that challenge her cognitive abilities such as Sudoku, and she watches the television news every night to keep up with the most recent occurrences in the world.

One may argue that the combination of high educational level, moderately active lifestyle, and a balanced diet have enhanced Mrs. M's cognitive reserve. However, the fact that her husband, who has the same educational level of Mrs. M and was exposed basically to the same environmental factors during the last 50 years, suggests that innate characteristics should be further explored to better understand "reserve" in the face of AD pathology.

As a final remark, it is important to mention that according to current appropriate criteria, the clinical use of amyloid PET is not recommended to asymptomatic individuals given the absence of an effective preventive therapy. Thus, although one might argue that the information regarding the neuroimaging results could encourage the patient presented here either to consider to move in the future to an assisted residence or to volunteer to a preventive clinical trial, the benefits and risks associated with this disclosure remain unclear. Rather than the mere presence of brain pathophysiology, this case illustrates that progression to dementia depends highly on other factors such as brain vulnerability as well as mechanisms underlying the so-called reserve. Therefore, the study of asymptomatic individuals such as the case presented here will make determining the underpinnings of vulnerability or resilience possible and help to elucidate the importance of disclosure biomarker results in asymptomatic subjects in the context of future disease-modifying therapies.

5.9 Take-Home Message

Preclinical stages are characterized by disease pathophysiology in the absence of symptoms.

Further Reading

Katzman R, Aronson M, Fuld P, et al. Development of dementing illnesses in an 80-year-old volunteer cohort. *Ann Neurol.* 1989;25:317–324.

Scarmeas N, Stern Y. Cognitive reserve and lifestyle. *J Clin Exp Neuropsychol.* 2003;25(5):625–633.

Stern Y. What is cognitive reserve? Theory and research application of the reserve concept. *J Int Neuropsychol Soc.* 2002;8(3):448–460.

Stern Y. Cognitive reserve and Alzheimer disease. *Alzheimer Dis Assoc Disord.* 2006; 20(2):112–117.

Wu YT, Teale J, Matthews FE, et al. Lifestyle factors, cognitive reserve, and cognitive function: results from the Cognitive Function and Ageing Study Wales, a population-based cohort. *Lancet.* 2016;388: S114.

A Challenging Thesis

Pedro Rosa-Neto, Monica Shin, Tharick A. Pascoal, Mira Chamoun,
Jean-Paul Soucy, Sarinporn Manitsirikul, and Serge Gauthier

6.1 Main Complaint

An 80-year-old man came to the consultation with problems in writing a thesis.

6.2 Clinical History

This retired teacher came alone to the first consultation mentioning that he was having difficulties writing a thesis at a local educational institution. He described that his thoughts were not as clear as before and that he struggled to focus on a specific idea during the process of drafting his thesis. As an example, he experienced difficulties in articulating his thoughts into meaningful sentences and noticed delays in finding words to appropriately complete them. Indeed, similar word-finding difficulties became apparent, particularly during conversations with his peers and advisor. Regarding memory, he mentioned that, in order to prevent problems, he became more dependent on his agenda, calendars, and notes as compared to a few years ago. In spite of these symptoms, he was capable of taking all the courses and requirements for graduating. He denied problems related to drawing abilities, visual problems, anxiety, or depression. He was managing his financial affairs, and he was driving safely. At home, he used to help his wife with simple tasks such as setting the table and doing the dishes. He denied past medical history of neurological conditions, including brain trauma, stroke, or neuropsychiatric conditions. On his first examination, he obtained 27 on the Montreal Cognitive Assessment (MoCA) (−3 on delayed recall), 29 on the Mini-Mental State Examination (MMSE) (−1 on copy design), and 18 on the Frontal Assessment Battery (FAB). The rest of the neurological examination was normal. His MRI showed few white matter hyperintensities (Fazekas = 1) and hippocampal atrophy (Scheltens = 3). He had an inconclusive [18F]fluorodeoxyglucose (FDG) PET scan, not fully compatible with Alzheimer's disease (AD).

Nearly 5 years later, after a successful thesis defense, this man returned to the consultation, now accompanied by his spouse, describing exacerbation of previous symptoms. He also started noticing inability to maintain the thread of a conversation as he used to do previously. In fact, he stopped speaking in public, due to frequent pauses since words were not becoming available while speaking the way they used to previously. He continued to use his computer but not as fast as before. His wife remarked that he started forgetting names of friends and familiar people. She also highlighted the patient's difficulties to retain the content of conversations. The wife also noticed some degree of social withdrawal, possibly due to language difficulties. Apart from reduced motivation to conduct his tasks at home, the wife denied significant behavioral changes such as hallucinations, delusions, mood alterations, repetitive behaviors, or reduced empathy. His wife and other family members started to manage the patient's financial affairs. The patient and his wife denied the presence of disorientation, motor symptoms, or falls.

6.3 General History

The patient had 21 years of education with a doctoral degree. He was taking daily doses of vitamin B12, ramipril 10 mg, atorvastatin, and insulin.

6.4 Examination

On his second visit, the physical examination was unremarkable. During the mental status exam, he was cooperative, attentive, and responsive and oriented in time and space. However, his Clinical Dementia Rating (CDR) was 1, MoCA progressed to 19/30, and the MMSE was 24/30, with normal immediate recall. The reverse order tests were abnormal. He made a few mistakes on the serial 7. Copy and clock drawing were normal. Anterograde memory evoked by a delayed recall showed deficits, which were partially corrected by cueing. Judgment and abstract thoughts were appropriated. The language assessment revealed an abnormal Boston naming test score of 6/25. The semantic fluency was reduced; however, the phonemic-letter fluency (FAS) was normal. The Boston Aphasia Examination test showed normal reading and comprehension. The rest of the neurological examination was normal. A second MRI ruled

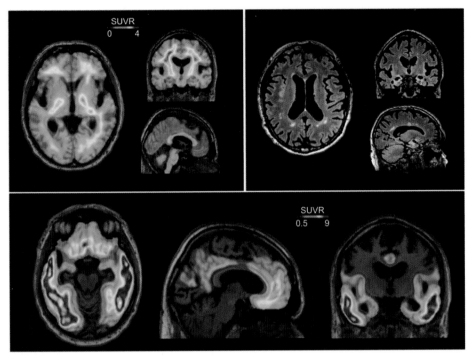

Figure 6.1 Top left shows a negative amyloid imaging conducted with the imaging agent [^{18}F]NAV4694, revealing no cortical or subcortical amyloid deposits. Top right shows FLAIR sequence with multiple white matter hyperintensities with some degree of confluency on the posterior horn of the lateral ventricle along with an atrophy of the hippocampus (Schelten's scale 3–4). Lower image shows positive tau imaging conducted with the imaging agent [^{18}F]MK-6240, revealing abnormal tau deposits on the temporal cortex L > R; orbitofrontal cortex, entorhinal cortices, hippocampus, and amygdala.

out brain infarcts and confirmed white matter hyper-intensities (Fazekas = 1) and mild progression of hippocampal atrophy (Scheltens = 3–4). A second [^{18}F]FDG PET scan showed mild reduction on the FDG uptake in the posterior cingulate, suggesting early AD. Amyloid PET was negative and tau PET was positive on the temporal lobe (mesial, basal, and neocortical) precuneous, inferior parietal cortex, orbitofrontal cortex, and amygdala (Braak stage 5; see Figure 6.1).

6.5 Family History

The family history was negative for dementias but positive for cerebrovascular disease on the maternal side.

6.6 Follow-Up

This patient developed significant neuropsychiatric symptoms characterized by anxiety and irritability that responded well to small doses of quetiapine (25 mg QD).

6.7 Diagnosis

The absence of signal in the amyloid PET and the positivity of tau PET support an in vivo diagnosis of neurofibrillary tangle predominant dementia (-NFTPD). It is challenging to assess the contributions of cerebrovascular disease to this clinical presentation given the age at onset, the multidomain cognitive presentation, the presence of risk factors of cerebrovascular diseases, and the presence of some MRI features suggestive of small vessels diseases.

6.8 Discussion

NFTPD was first described by Ulrich and colleagues, as a sporadic subtype of progressive dementia found in nearly 5% of very old demented subjects. This clinicopathological entity is characterized by an abundant allocortical and isocortex neurofibrillary pathology, usually extending to Braak stages III and IV, in the absence of mature amyloid plaques. However, diffuse plaques or mild cerebral amyloid antipathy (CAA) might be detectable in up to 25% of these cases. If present, subcortical tau pathology is mainly restricted to the amygdala, nucleus basalis of Meynert, and locus coeruleus. Although presenting similarities with AD, NFTPD seems insensitive to APOE4 genotype. Despite more neuropsychiatric manifestations, NFTPD cognitive impairment seems less severe and the age at onset manifests later (>80 years of age).

Similar to NFTPD, the recently introduced concept of primary age-related tauopathy (PART) describes a rather common pathological finding in the brains of elderly individuals with neurofibrillary tangles that is indistinguishable from those of AD, in the absence of amyloid plaques. In PART, the neurofibrillary pathology is mostly restricted to structures in the medial temporal lobe, basal forebrain, brainstem, and olfactory areas (bulb and cortex). As PART cases range from normal to mild amnestic cognitive impairment, the designation of "NFT-only dementia" or "NFTPD" cases seem inappropriate. Although sharing common clinicopathological features, it remains debatable whether NFTPD, PART, and AD constitute the spectrum of a single disease mechanism.

This case illustrates a late-onset cognitive syndrome beginning in a highly educated individual, who had his first symptoms in the context of an intellectually challenging life experience. The initial presentation of the symptoms in this patient was observable nearly exclusively in a situation of high intellectual demand and imperceptible for family members. Specifically, one might claim a multi-domain presentation characterized by a minor anterograde memory deficit component and a major world-searching component. The involvement of naming and other semantic deficits with the disease progression was noticeable. These initial symptoms steadily progressed with a late expression of neuropsychiatric symptoms such as anxiety and irritability. The rate of progression presented in this case is typical to cases with high cognitive reserve.

From the pathophysiological perspective, these clinical symptoms occurred in the context of brain atrophy and mild metabolic deficits localizing in areas of the posterior cingulate, frontal, and temporal cortices as well as the presence of neurofibrillary tangles (paired helical filament), however, without amyloid as detected by PET imaging. Together, this clinico-pathophysiological presentation supports a diagnosis of NFTPD.

The in vivo diagnosis of PART or NFTPD is in its infancy; it has only been possible due to advances in neuroimaging. The in vivo diagnosis of PART or NFTPD might help on the description of this neglected clinical entity, possibly, playing a role in the patient enrollment of clinical trials involving disease-modifying therapies targeting amyloid pathology. Assuming that the tau imaging agent utilized here is selective for combined 3 and 4 R tau isoforms of paired helical conformations, one might claim that the imaging findings presented differ from carriers of MAPT R406W mutations, who might show temporal lobe predominant tauopathy with similar features to NFTPD.

The concept that multiple pathologies coexist in the brain of dementia patients has been corroborated by numerous cohorts. Possibly, cerebrovascular disease might play a role in patients with older ages and risk factors for cerebrovascular disease. In fact, current MRI techniques fail to reveal microscopic vascular alterations present in geriatric populations. Both TDP43 pathology or hippocampal sclerosis are also present in elderly patients and constitute a possible comorbidity in this case, particularly in patients with semantic profile.

The management of PART or NFTPD cases remains empirical and symptomatic, and possibly future clinical trials or personalized medicine approaches might reveal the optimal management of these individuals. Possibly, the management risk factors for cerebrovascular disease in those individuals with diabetes, hypertension, and dyslipidemia would have an impact on the care of these individuals. Cognitive stimulation, diet, and physical exercise also might play a role in the management of these cases.

6.9 Take-Home Messages

1. A small fraction of the population with dementia show a biomarker profile characterized as positive for tau and negative for amyloid scan. This clinico-pathophysiological entity supports the clinicopathological concept of NFTPD.

2. Further studies focusing on the natural history, genetics, and therapeutic management should be conducted in order to better manage these cases. In fact, 90+ is the fastest growing segment of the population in some countries.

3. Tau imaging might be clinically relevant for differentiating NFTPD and PART from frontotemporal dementia cases.

Further Reading

Attems J, Jellinger KA. Amyloid and tau: neither chicken nor egg but two partners in crime! *Acta Neuropathol.* 2013;126: 619–621.

Braak H, Del Tredici K. Are cases with tau pathology occurring in the absence of Aβ deposits part of the AD-related pathological process? *Acta Neuropathol.* 2014;128:767–772.

Crary JF, Trojanowski JQ, Schneider JA, et al. Primary age-related tauopathy (PART): a common pathology associated with human aging. *Acta Neuropathol.* 2014;128:755–766.

Delacourte A. The natural and molecular history of Alzheimer's disease. *J Alzheimer Dis.* 2006;9:187–194.

Jellinger KA. Complex tauopathies versus tangle predominant dementia. *Acta Neuropathol.* 2011;122(4):515.

Jellinger KA, Attems J. Neurofibrillary tangle-predominant dementia: comparison with classical Alzheimer disease. *Acta Neuropathol.* 2006;113: 107–117.

Jellinger KA, Alafuzoff I, Attems J, et al. PART, a distinct tauopathy, different from classical sporadic Alzheimer disease. *Acta Neuropathol.* 2015;129: 757–762.

Josephs KA, Murray ME, Tosakulwong N, et al. Tau aggregation influences cognition and hippocampal atrophy in the absence of beta-amyloid: a clinico-imaging-pathological study of primary age-related tauopathy (PART). *Acta Neuropathol.* 2017;133:705–715.

Masahito Y. Senile dementia of the neurofibrillary tangle type (tangle-only dementia): neuropathological criteria and clinical guidelines for diagnosis. *Neuropathol.* 2003;23:311–317.

Weller RO, Hawkes CA, Carare RO, Hardy J. Does the difference between PART and Alzheimer's disease lie in the age-related changes in cerebral arteries that trigger the accumulation of Aβ and propagation of tau? *Acta Neuropathol.* 2015;129:763–766.

The Forgetful Golfer

Marlee Parsons, Monica Shin, Tharick A. Pascoal, Mira Chamoun,
Joseph Therriault, Jean-Paul Soucy, Serge Gauthier, and Pedro Rosa-Neto

7.1 Primary Problem

Decline in memory function.

7.2 Clinical History

A 65-year-old retired administrative assistant was referred by her family doctor to investigate reduced memory function. Her partner was also present during the consultation. On his referral letter, the family doctor mentioned a decline in the patient cognition, without abnormalities on the laboratory tests or brain CT. During the consultation, the patient described difficulties in keeping track of conversations when she was playing golf. She was definitively more dependent on her notes and on her smartphone to remember appointments out of her routine. She mentioned a lack of attention and memory lapses were causing some level of embarrassment during her social activities. She also noticed that she was getting easily fatigued and not as fast as before in performing her domestic duties. Although the partner expressed some concerns regarding the patient's emotional independence, she confirmed that the patient remains independent regarding personal and financial affairs.

7.3 General History

The patient had normal blood pressure, lipid profile, glycemia, and practiced daily exercises as a routine for many years. The couple followed a Mediterranean-like diet and there was no clinical history of recent sleep abnormalities and cardiovascular, respiratory, or urinary problems. From the neuropsychiatric perspective, there was no clinical history of disinhibition, reduced impulse control, substance-related disorders, stereotypical or ritualistic symptoms, hallucinations, or delusions.

7.4 Examination

The blood pressure and the cardiac rhythm were normal, as well as the carotid auscultation. Her MoCA score was 23/30 (impairment confined to delayed recall). From a cognitive perspective, she had a normal executive function as well as speed of processing, visual attention, working memory, and social cognition. The cranial nerves, reflexes, motor, cerebellar, and sensory examinations were normal. Her gait and stance were unremarkable.

7.5 Laboratory Tests

Laboratory tests were all normal. Apolipoprotein E genotype revealed that this patient was a double E4 carrier. The patient decided to engage in research protocols and had amyloid and tau scans conducted with [18F]AZD4694 and [18F]MK6240, respectively (Figure 7.1a and b). The amyloid scan revealed high uptake of amyloid in the precuneus, anterior and posterior cingulate, inferior parietal, basolateral temporal, and occipital cortices. Tau images also reveal abnormal uptake in the mesial temporal cortex, lateral temporal cortex, anterior and posterior cingulate, as well as prefrontal cortices in a topology compatible with Braak stages 4–5. Brain magnetic resonance imaging (MRI) showed a bilateral reduction of volumes in the hippocampus (R > L; Scheltens scale = 4). No acute ischemic changes were seen in DWI or ADC.

7.6 Family History

The patient's mother died with complications of Alzheimer's disease (AD) at the age of 81 years. She had two out of five maternal siblings affected by AD. There was no information regarding the paternal side of her family. None of her younger brothers were affected.

7.7 Follow-Up

Nearly 2 years later, the patient scored 23/30 (memory and serial 7s) on MoCA. The patient now needs her partner's assistance to manage her financial affairs. She started with cholinesterase inhibitors, and a few months later, she decided to volunteer in a clinical trial with an experimental

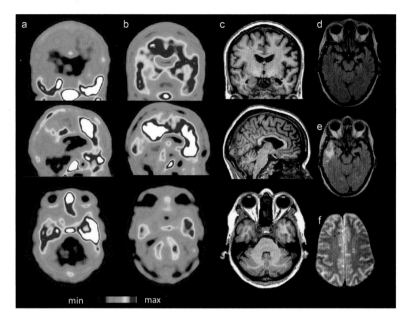

Figure 7.1 Images represent in vivo quantification of brain amyloid and tau aggregates obtained using the [^{18}F]MK6240 (a) and [^{18}F]AZD4694 PET imaging agents (b). T1-weighted structural MRI (c) shown at the same levels as the PET images indicate the brain regions affected by amyloid and tau deposition in this patient as well as right hippocampal atrophy (c, red arrow). FLAIR MRI sequence before (d) and after the anti-amyloid therapy (e) shows the hyperintensity (ARIA, e) in the left temporal neocortex (red arrow) suggestive of vasogenic edema. (f) Frontal area with hypointensity observed on the GRET2* sequence (red arrow).

therapy for AD. In a subsequent visit, she mentioned that, unfortunately, she decided to withdraw from the study due to the presence of a side effect detected by the safety MRIs. A new MRI confirmed the presence of increased white matter signal in the right temporal lobe (Figure 7.1e) in the fluid-attenuated inversion recovery (FLAIR) sequences. There were also various 1–3 mm dark spots in the frontal and temporal regions on the susceptibility sequence (GRE T2*; Figure 7.1f).

7.8 Diagnosis

The diagnosis of the dementia syndrome of this patient according to the 2018 NIA-AA research criteria is Alzheimer's disease with dementia. Biomarkers support this diagnosis. As shown in Figure 7.1, positive amyloid and tau positron emission tomography (PET) imaging confirmed the presence of AD pathophysiology. Hippocampal atrophy provided evidence of neurodegeneration in the MRI[1] in accordance to the 2011 NIA-AA criteria, which states the diagnosis is AD dementia with evidence of the AD pathophysiological process.[2] The adverse events emergent during the clinical trial were amyloid-related imaging abnormalities (ARIA). Imaging findings support the presence of

vasogenic edema (ARIA-E) hemosiderin deposition (ARIA-H).

7.9 Discussion

This case describes a 65-year-old patient homozygous for the apolipoprotein E4 polymorphism with a progressive cognitive syndrome dominated by anterograde memory deficits. This patient had a significant adverse event associated with an amyloid-lowering agent in the context of a clinical trial. As this patient participated in various research protocols, it was possible to describe this case using the recent research diagnostic criteria based on the presence of amyloid (A) and tau (T) aggregates as well neurodegeneration (N) measured via biomarkers (Tables 7.1 and 7.2).

The information of amyloid and tau imaging available in this case describes a patient with complete AD pathophysiology (A+T+N+) with MCI who subsequently progressed to AD (A+T+N+) with dementia (Tables 7.1 and 7.2). Although this new diagnostic criterion brings more precision to the diagnosis of dementia, one should be aware that it cannot rule out the presence of commodities with other protein aggregates such as Lewy body or TDP-43.

Table 7.1 Alzheimer's disease clinical staging according to 2018 National Institute on Aging (NIA) at National Institutes of Health (NIH) and the Alzheimer's Association published revised guidelines (NIA-AA)

Clinical stage	Syndromal stage	Clinical features
1	Cognitively unimpaired	Cognitive symptoms: absent Cognition: normal range Functional decline: absent
2	Cognitively unimpaired	Cognitive symptoms: present Cognition: normal range Functional decline: absent
3	Mild cognitive impairment	Cognitive decline: present Cognition: normal present Functional decline: present but patient remains autonomous
4	Dementia (mild)	Cognitive decline: present Cognition: multidomain deficits Functional decline: loss of autonomy and requires occasional assistance with daily activities
5	Dementia (moderated)	Cognitive decline: present Cognition: multidomain deficits Functional decline: requires frequent assistance with daily activities
6	Dementia (severe)	Cognitive decline: present Cognition: multidomain deficits Functional decline: requires complete assistance with daily activities

Given the lack of therapies for AD, the clinical utility of the new classification remains limited. However, in the context of clinical trials, this new classification better defines stages of AD across its entire spectrum and constitutes an important advance for drug development programs and observational research. The new classification incorporated the rapid advances in the field of biomarkers such as the various *in vivo* post-mortem validation studies. Overall, this framework consolidates cerebrospinal fluid and PET imaging as surrogates for amyloid and tau neuropathology. In addition, the same framework recognizes [18F]fluorodeoxyglucose PET, MRI, and total tau (t-tau) as proxies for neurodegeneration rather than specific diseases processes.

Interventions modifying amyloid in the brain bring the risk of amyloid-related imaging abnormalities (ARIA).[3,4,5,6] The term ARIA incorporates brain edema or effusions (ARIA-E) linked to MR signal alterations thought to reflect vasogenic edema or other related extravasated fluid phenomena. ARIA-hemosiderin deposition (ARIA-H) refers to the 1–2 mm MR signal hypodensities attributable to microhemorrhage or hemosiderosis. The comorbidity between ARIA-H and ARIA-E is frequent.

The diagnosis of ARIA-E requires FLAIR acquisitions and two-dimensional T2*-GRE for identifying ARIA-H. Carriers of ARIA brain abnormalities frequently remain asymptomatic and are mostly diagnosed on the bases of safety MRIs conducted during clinical trials. However, patients with ARIA might manifest clinical symptoms such as headaches, confusion, visual disturbance, and gait difficulties. The presence of apolipoprotein E4 homozygotes, white matter hyperintensities, or microhemorrhages is related to higher risk of developing ARIA. Imaging findings associated with ARIA might be similar to cerebral amyloid angiopathy. Further studies are necessary to determine the natural history and prevention of these brain abnormalities.

7.10 Take-Home Messages

1. Amyloid-related imaging abnormalities (ARIA) constitute a potential side effect associated with multiple therapeutic strategies targeting to lower amyloid-β burden of AD.

2. ARIA encompasses hyperintensities on the FLAIR as well as signal hypointensities on the GRE/T2* sequences, which might indicate vasogenic edema (ARIA-E) and hemosiderin deposits (ARIA-H), including microhemorrhage and superficial siderosis.

3. Safety MRIs constitute an important tool for assessing adverse reaction to anti-amyloid therapies.

Table 7.2 2018 NI-AA Alzheimer's disease cognitive staging with all possible biomarker profiles

	A	T	N	Cognitively unimpaired	Mild cognitive impairment	Dementia
					Cognitive stage	
Biomarker Profile	−	−	−	Normal AD biomarkers, cognitively unimpaired	Normal AD biomarkers with MCI	Normal AD biomarkers with dementia
	+	−	−	Preclinical Alzheimer's pathologic change	Alzheimer's pathologic change with MCI	Alzheimer's pathologic change with dementia
	+	+	−	Preclinical AD	AD with MCI (prodromal AD)	AD with dementia
	+	+	+			
	+	−	+	Alzheimer's and concomitant suspected non-Alzheimer's pathologic change, cognitively unimpaired	Alzheimer's and concomitant suspected non-Alzheimer's pathologic change with MCI	Alzheimer's and concomitant suspected non-Alzheimer's pathologic change with dementia
	−	+	−	Non-Alzheimer's pathologic change, cognitively unimpaired	Non-Alzheimer's pathologic change with MCI	Non-Alzheimer's pathologic change with dementia
	−	−	+			
	−	+	+			

AD, Alzheimer disease; MCI, mild cognitive impairment.
Adapted from Jack et al. (2018)[1]

References

1. Jack CR Jr, Bennett DA, Blennow K, et al. NIA-AA Research Framework: toward a biological definition of Alzheimer's disease. *Alzheimers Dement.* 2018;14 (4):535–562. doi: 10.1016/j. jalz.2018.02.018.

2. Mo JJ, Li JY, Yang Z, Liu Z, Feng JS. Efficacy and safety of anti-amyloid-β immunotherapy for Alzheimer's disease: a systematic review and network meta-analysis. *Ann Clin Transl Neurol.* 2017;4(12):931–942. doi: 10.1002/acn3.469.

3. Barakos J, Sperling R, Salloway S, et al. MR imaging features of amyloid-related imaging abnormalities. *AJNR Am J Neuroradiol.* 2013;34 (10):1958–1965. doi: 10.3174/ajnr. A3500.

4. Sperling R, Salloway S, Brooks DJ, et al. Amyloid-related imaging abnormalities in patients with Alzheimer's disease treated with bapineuzumab: a retrospective analysis. *Lancet Neurol.* 2012;11 (3):241–249. doi: 10.1016/S1474-4422(12)70015-7.

5. Sperling RA, Jack CR Jr, Black SE, et al. Amyloid-related imaging abnormalities in amyloid-modifying therapeutic trials: recommendations from the Alzheimer's Association Research Roundtable Workgroup. *Alzheimers Dement.* 2011;7 (4):367–385. doi: 10.1016/j. jalz.2011.05.2351.

6. McKhann GM, Knopman DS, Chertkow H, et al. The diagnosis of dementia due to Alzheimer's disease: recommendations from the National Institute on Aging-Alzheimer's Association workgroups on diagnostic guidelines for Alzheimer's disease. *Alzheimers Dement.* 2011;7 (3):263–269. doi: 10.1016/j. jalz.2011.03.005.

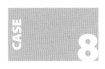

The Innapropriate Pedagogue

Leandro Boson Gambogi, Leonardo Cruz de Souza,
Henrique Cerqueira Guimarães, and Paulo Caramelli

8.1 Clinical History – Main Complaint

ALLG is a 57-year-old married woman, with 15 years of schooling (graduated in pedagogy).

At the age of 50 her husband noted that ALLG became more participative in church. Once restrained and timid, ALLG began to use the microphone to preach during church services, manifesting an unprecedented religious fanaticism. She suddenly quit eating meat and only accepted what she considered "healthy food." She started to collect stuff without obvious actual utility, including plastic bags and empty butter pots and soda cans. She also engaged in repetitively tapping on things (tables, chairs) without any reasonable purpose. Her abilities to deal with administrative and financial tasks, housekeeping, and cooking became impaired. Before neurological evaluation at our unit, the patient had consulted a psychiatrist, who established the diagnosis of depression.

ALLG became progressively more inappropriate, especially in social events, when she started embarrassing her family relatives. ALLG would easily call someone she barely knew as a sinner and order the person to seek the Lord. However, she kept working until the age 53, when she got her first medical disability due to behavioral and personality changes, and difficulty in planning her daily activities.

Despite her husband's compelling complaints, ALLG made no remarks regarding her condition during first evaluation, except for insomnia. She denied all her husband's descriptions.

8.2 General History

ALLG was born in the countryside of Minas Gerais, Brazil. She graduated in pedagogy from University of São Paulo, where she lived until she turned 30 years old. Then she went back to her hometown and worked as a pedagogue until her retirement. ALLG is married and has one son.

The patient was previously healthy, with no comorbidities. She had no history of developmental learning or language problems, previous psychiatric or neurological problems.

8.3 Family History

There were six cases of early-onset dementia in her family, including her brother, father, grandfather, and three uncles. Her husband could not provide clinical details on their presentation but stressed they presented remarkable behavioral changes.

8.4 Examination

8.4.1 Neurological Exam

Her neurological exam was normal, without motor or sensory deficits or balance impairment. Primitive reflexes (grasp and palmomental) were the only detected alterations.

8.4.2 Neuropsychological and Functional Assessment

ALLG scored 26/30 in the Mini-Mental State Examination (MMSE), 9/18 in the Frontal Assessment Battery, 17 in the phonemic verbal fluency (FAS test), 13 in category fluency test (animals), and 6 in the delayed recall in the visual memory test from the Brief Cognitive Screening Battery.[1] She underwent an evaluation of social cognition with the Brazilian short version of the Social and Emotional Assessment.[2] This exam disclosed severe deficits in emotion recognition of Ekman faces (score 15/35) and theory of mind assessed by the faux pas test (score 12/40).

The functional assessment showed impaired abilities. She scored 10/30 in the Functional Activities Questionnaire (FAQ)[3] and 43% in Frontotemporal Dementia Rating Scale (FRS).[4]

Neuropsychological tests pointed to a mild impairment in executive functions and performance at lower limits in other abilities (Table 8.1). Of note, she also had severe deficits in social cognition tests. According to her husband, she was independent for basic activities of daily living but not for instrumental ones.

8.4.3 Neuroimaging Findings

Brain MRI (Figure 8.1) shows severe anterior right temporal atrophy, including frontoinsular region. There was mild atrophy in left temporal lobe and in

Table 8.1 Performance on neuropsychological assessments

Mini-Mental State Exam	Time orientation (/5)	5
	Space orientation (/5)	5
	Repetition (/3)	3
	Attention/Calculation (/5)	3
		1
	Recall (/3)	8
	Language (/8)	1
	Copy draw (/1)	26
	Total (/30)	
Episodic Memory	Incidental (/10)	5
	Immediate (/10)	6
	Learning (/10)	8
	Delayed Recall – 5 min (/10)	6
	Recognition (/10)	10
Frontal Assessment Battery	Conceptualization (/3)	1
	Lexical fluency (/3)	2
	Motor programming (/3)	1
		3
	Conflicting instruction (/3)	1
	Inhibitory control (/3)	1
		9
	Environmental autonomy (/3)	
	Total (/18)	
Verbal Fluency	Animals	13
	FAS	17
Social Cognition	Recognition of facial emotion (/35)	15
	Theory of mind (faux pas test) (/40)	20

frontal lobes, especially medial frontal (red circle). Severe anterior right temporal atrophy, including frontoinsular region. There was mild atrophy in left temporal lobe and in frontal lobes, especially medial frontal (red circle). Posterior regions were preserved. There were no focal or vascular lesions.

8.4.4 Biomarkers and Genetic Analysis

The patient also underwent lumbar puncture in order to investigate cerebrospinal fluid (CSF) biomarkers related to Alzheimer's disease (AD). The analysis did not show a CSF AD profile (Aβ42 = 945.69 pg/mL, Tau = 245.03 pg/mL, p-Tau = 33.16 pg/mL).

Since ALLG had a family history compatible with an autosomal dominant inheritance, her DNA was extracted from peripheral blood leukocytes using previously described methods.[5] Sequencing data were analyzed with Mutation Surveyor v3.2 (SoftGenetics)[6] and a mutation of the TARDBP gene, located on chromosome 1, was identified (genetic analysis conducted by Dr. Leonel T. Takada at the University of São Paulo, Brazil).

8.5 Diagnosis

Based on the clinical, neuropsychological, and neuroimaging data a diagnosis of probable behavioral variant frontotemporal dementia (bvFTD) was established. The definitive diagnosis was confirmed by genetic analysis.

8.6 Follow-Up

The patient was submitted to symptomatic pharmacological treatment. Trazodone was chosen, due to the evidence of benefits.[7] After 2 weeks the patient was evaluated with improvement in repetitive movements and hoarding. Disinhibition was still an issue and doses of trazodone were gradually increased until 300 mg/day.

Two months after use of trazodone on maximum dosage, the patient was putting herself in risk, walking

Figure 8.1 Brain MRI.

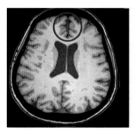
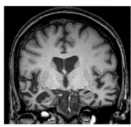
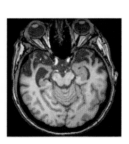

from the country house to the city by herself, being lost from the family, talking loudly during church, and refusing treatment. After a failed trial with quetiapine, risperidone (1 mg/day) was initiated.[8]

The patient kept herself stable for a year. When she tried to misrepresent a document in doctor's name in order to stop treatment (Figure 8.2), risperidone was increased to 2 mg/day and then to 3 mg/day. ALLG became severely apathetic, with overt extrapyramidal symptoms. However, drug regimen was maintained due to severity of her behavioral symptoms, and 1 year later it was reduced.

Almost 7 years after symptoms onset and 3 years after our first evaluation, the patient remains on trazodone (300 mg/day) and risperidone (1 mg/day), and also duloxetine (30 mg/day). She presents severe apathy, puerility, and mild disinhibition, with no hoarding or dietary changes. Regardless of her clinical presentation, she is still partially independent for basic activities of daily living.

8.7 Discussion

ALLG's symptoms depict a very typical case of bvFTD, a clinical syndrome characterized by progressive behavioral and personality changes related to atrophy of the frontal and temporal brain regions.[9] Those dramatic changes in personality and behavioral traits may occur in the absence of obvious cognitive impairment, as illustrated in the case above.

FTD and its variants account for about 15% of primary neurodegenerative diseases, and is considered the second cause of early-onset dementia. The behavioral variant is the most frequent presentation, being responsible for more than half of the cases.[10]

Previously recognized under the concept of Pick's disease,[11] FTD diagnostic criteria were first developed by a consensus of researchers from Lund, Sweden, and Manchester, England, in 1994.[12] The criteria were subsequently refined by an international consensus in

DECLARAÇÃO MEDICA

Prezado Senhores da Igreja Adventista do 7 dia declaramos que a Paciente Ana   está ótima e não precisa tomar mais remédio, se precisar tomar remédio para dormir pode procurar outro Médico. Pode a deixar ela participar da sua igreja Cantando, orando e pregando a palavra de Deus

Ela está liberada para dirigir o carro. Você precisa considerar ela com muito carinho. Declaramos que ela esta curada.

Dr.

PSIQUIATRIA

CRMmg

CONTROLE 6814174

Belo Horizonte   02 de Outubro de 2015

Figure 8.2 Patient's misrepresented document.
Figure 8.2 translation: "Dear Seventh-day Adventist Church Sir we declare that Patient A... is great and does not need to take any more medicines, if she needs to take sleeping pills she could seek another Physician. You can let her participate in church services, Singing, praying and preaching the word of God. She is free to drive a car. You must consider her with great affection. We declare she is cured." This is an *ipsis litteris* translation of her letter including several grammar mistakes.

1998[13] and included a set of "core" and "supportive" features to the diagnosis. The clinical framework for the bvFTD diagnosis were revised in 2011,[14] which resulted in diagnostic criteria sensitivity improvement. Since then, a bvFTD phenotype can be verified according to the presence of progressive behavioral and/or cognition deterioration, in addition to at least three out of six possible core symptoms: (1) social disinhibition; (2) apathy; (3) loss of sympathy or empathy; (4) perseverative, stereotyped, or compulsive behavior; (5) hyperorality and dietary changes; (6) a neuropsychological profile characterized by executive dysfunction, with relative preservation of episodic memory and visuospatial abilities. The diagnosis is considered probable when frontal and/or anterior temporal atrophy is found on structural neuroimaging, or otherwise functional neuroimaging techniques disclose perfusion/metabolism deficits in the aforementioned topography. A definitive diagnosis of bvFTD is reserved only to cases with histopathological confirmation and/or presence of a known pathogenic genetic mutation.

In parallel to advances in clinical characterization, mutations associated with the FTD have been identified since 1998, when mutations in the microtubule-associated protein tau (MAPT) gene on chromosome 17 were first recognized in families with FTD and parkinsonism.[15] Since then, 10 other genes have been associated with FTD spectrum disorders. In 2006, the second FTD-related gene on chromosome 17 was discovered: mutations in the progranulin (GRN) gene accounted for even more FTD cases than mutations in MAPT. In 2011, an expanded hexanucleotide repeat in a noncoding region of the chromosome 9 open reading frame 72 (C9orf72) gene was identified as a cause of FTD, amyotrophic lateral sclerosis (ALS), and FTD associated with motor neuron disease (MND), by two independent research groups. Along with C9orf72, mutations in GRN and MAPT are the most commonly identified in FTD cohorts.[16] Surprisingly, a single genetic mutation was found to account for completely different clinical pictures and also for variable neuroimaging phenotypes, even within the same family.[17]

Other uncommon mutations have been identified in the valosin-containing protein (VCP) gene, which cause inclusion body myopathy with Paget disease of bone and FTD; in the charged multivesicular body protein 2B (CHMP2B) gene, involved in the endosomal–lysosomal pathway; and also mutations in the fused sarcoma (FUS), dynactin (DCTN1), sequestosome 1 (SQSTM1), colony-stimulating factor 1 receptor (CFS1R), triggering receptor expressed on myeloid cells (TREM2), ubiquilin-2 (UBQLN2), and heterogeneous nuclear ribonucleoprotein A2B1 (hnRNPA2B1) genes.

The TARDBP gene, located on chromosome 1, is responsible for encoding the TDP-43 (transactive response DNA-binding protein, 43 kDa), a major pathological protein found in ubiquitin inclusions, which are present in almost half of FTLD cases. Mutations in TARDBP gene usually give rise to an ALS phenotype, but also – although infrequently – can cause FTD-MND or bvFTD clinical presentations. The bvFTD was the most frequently found phenotype in a recent large series study of patients with TARDBP mutations presenting with FTD.[18] Common behavioral features of FTD associated with TARDBP are dietary restriction, repetitive behavior, and impairment of social-emotional cognition,[19] such as ALLG case. Her neuroimaging findings depicted a predominant right temporal involvement, which stands in accordance with a recent report on TARDBP mutation carriers.[19] This neuroimaging characteristic can be associated with two main clinical pictures: bvFTD and right FTD temporal variant. In the latter, patients present overt prosopagnosia and language impairment,[20] which were absent in ALLG presentation.

In general, according to studies using voxel-based morphometry analysis through magnetic resonance imaging (MRI), the mainly affected areas correspond to the medial frontal lobe – particularly the cingulate gyrus, the medial orbitofrontal, and frontopolar portions – in addition to frontoinsular and temporal regions.[9] Temporal lobes are especially affected in behavioral presentations, particularly the inferopolar areas.

There are no disease-modifying therapies for any of the FTD underlying diseases. Treatment is focused on symptom management and providing support for patients, families, and caregivers. Selective serotonin reuptake inhibitors[21-23] and trazodone[7] are commonly used and may be beneficial for behavioral symptoms, including disinhibition, hyperorality, and stereotyped and ritualistic behaviors.

The prognosis of bvFTD is ominous, with a median survival of 8.7 years ($\pm$1.2 years).[24] Nonetheless, recent reports have documented slowly progressive presentations, sometimes with 20 years of survival.[25,26]

Patients and caregivers may be better managed by multidisciplinary teams, which could better address the complex and multifactorial demands (behavioral, cognitive, functional, legal, nutritional, mobility, swallowing) those patients usually present.[27]

Acknowledgments
Paulo Caramelli, MD, PhD, is funded by CNPq, Brazil. We thank Leonel T. Takada, MD, PhD, for the genetic analysis of this case.

References

1. Nitrini R, Lefevre BH, Mathias SC, et al. Neuropsychological tests of simple application for diagnosing dementia. *Arq Neuropsiquiatr.* 1994;52(4):457–465.

2. Bertoux M, Volle E, Funkiewiez A, et al. Social Cognition and Emotional Assessment (SEA) is a marker of medial and orbital frontal functions: a voxel-based morphometry study in behavioral variant of frontotemporal degeneration. *J Int Neuropsychol Soc.* 2012;18(6):972–985.

3. Pfeffer RI, Kurosaki TT, Harrah CH, Jr. et al. Measurement of functional activities in older adults in the community. *J Gerontol.* 1982;37(3):323–329.

4. Lima-Silva TB, Carvalho VA, Guimarães HC, Caramelli P, Balthazar M. Translation, cross-cultural adaptation and applicability of the Brazilian version of the Frontotemporal Dementia Rating Scale (FTD-FRS). *Dement Neuropsychol.* 2013;7:387–396.

5. Miller SA, Dykes DD, Polesky HF. A simple salting out procedure for extracting DNA from human nucleated cells. *Nucleic Acids Res.* 1988;16(3):1215.

6. Takada LT, Bahia VS, Guimaraes HC, et al. GRN and MAPT mutations in 2 Frontotemporal Dementia Research Centers in Brazil. *Alzheimer Dis Assoc Disord.* 2016;30(4):310–317.

7. Lebert F, Stekke W, Hasenbroekx C, Pasquier F. Frontotemporal dementia: a randomised, controlled trial with trazodone. *Dement Geriat Cogn Disord.* 2004;17(4):355–359.

8. Engelborghs S, Vloeberghs E, Le Bastard N, et al. The dopaminergic neurotransmitter system is associated with aggression and agitation in frontotemporal dementia. *Neurochem Int.* 2008;52(6):1052–1060.

9. Schroeter ML, Raczka K, Neumann J, von Cramon DY. Neural networks in frontotemporal dementia–a meta-analysis. *Neurobiol Aging.* 2008;29(3):418–426.

10. Onyike CU, Diehl-Schmid J. The epidemiology of frontotemporal dementia. *Int Rev psychiatry.* 2013;25(2):130–137.

11. Kertesz A. Frontotemporal dementia: a topical review. *Cognit Behav Neurol.* 2008;21(3):127–133.

12. The Lund and Manchester Groups. Clinical and neuropathological criteria for frontotemporal dementia. *J Neurol Neurosurg Psychiatry.* 1994;57(4):416–418.

13. Neary D, Snowden JS, Gustafson L, et al. Frontotemporal lobar degeneration: a consensus on clinical diagnostic criteria. *Neurology.* 1998;51(6):1546–1554.

14. Rascovsky K, Hodges JR, Knopman D, et al. Sensitivity of revised diagnostic criteria for the behavioural variant of frontotemporal dementia. *Brain.* 2011;134(Pt 9):2456–2477.

15. Rohrer JD, Guerreiro R, Vandrovcova J, et al. The heritability and genetics of frontotemporal lobar degeneration. *Neurology.* 2009;73(18):1451–1456.

16. Takada LT. The genetics of monogenic frontotemporal dementia. *Dement Neuropsychol.* 2015;9:219–229.

17. Benussi A, Padovani A, Borroni B. Phenotypic heterogeneity of monogenic frontotemporal dementia. *Front Aging neurosci.* 2015;7:171.

18. Caroppo P, Camuzat A, Guillot-Noel L, et al. Defining the spectrum of frontotemporal dementias associated with TARDBP mutations. *Neurol Genet.* 2016;2(3):e80.

19. Floris G, Borghero G, Cannas A, et al. Clinical phenotypes and radiological findings in frontotemporal dementia related to TARDBP mutations. *J Neurol.* 2015;262(2):375–384.

20. Kamminga J, Kumfor F, Burrell JR, et al. Differentiating between right-lateralised semantic dementia and behavioural-variant frontotemporal dementia: an examination of clinical characteristics and emotion processing. *J Neurol Neurosurg Psychiatry.* 2015;86(10):1082–1088.

21. Swartz JR, Miller BL, Lesser IM, Darby AL. Frontotemporal dementia: treatment response to serotonin selective reuptake inhibitors. *J Clin Psychiatry.* 1997;58(5):212–216.

22. Hughes LE, Rittman T, Regenthal R, Robbins TW, Rowe JB. Improving response inhibition systems in frontotemporal dementia with citalopram. *Brain.* 2015;138(Pt 7):1961–1975.

23. Chow TW, Mendez MF. Goals in symptomatic pharmacologic management of frontotemporal lobar degeneration. *Am J Alzheimers Dis Other Dement.* 2002;17(5):267–272.

24. Roberson ED, Hesse JH, Rose KD, et al. Frontotemporal dementia progresses to death faster than Alzheimer disease. *Neurology*. 2005;65(5):719–725.

25. Suhonen NM, Kaivorinne AL, Moilanen V, et al. Slowly progressive frontotemporal lobar degeneration caused by the C9ORF72 repeat expansion: a 20-year follow-up study. *Neurocase*. 2015;21(1):85–89.

26. Gomez-Tortosa E, Serrano S, de Toledo M, Perez-Perez J, Sainz MJ. Familial benign frontotemporal deterioration with C9ORF72 hexanucleotide expansion. *Alzheimers Dement*. 2014;10(5 Suppl):S284–S289.

27. Pressman PS, Miller BL. Diagnosis and management of behavioral variant frontotemporal dementia. *Biol Psychiatry*. 2014;75(7):574–581.

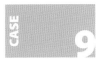

A 59-Year-Old Man with Weakness and Personality Changes

Parichita Choudhury, Gordon Jewett, Leonard Numerow,
Lawrence Korngut, and Gerald Pfeffer

9.1 Case

9.1.1 Clinical History – Main Complaint

A 59-year-old, right-hand-dominant man presented to the emergency department complaining that he could not move his right foot. Over the past month his right leg had become progressively weaker. He had difficulty climbing stairs and was frequently tripping over his right foot, which had resulted in more than one serious fall. During this period he felt a sensation of muscle tightness and frequent cramps in his right posterior thigh and lower leg.

In addition, the patient complained of poor memory and emotional lability. He was having difficulty remembering names of people he knew well, and had gotten lost in familiar places on several occasions. He reported irritability and frequent outbursts of anger, while his daughter noted rapid shifts from anger to tears.

9.1.2 General History

On detailed questioning the patient reported that he had been having difficulty walking for a few months. He described that his right foot would flop and smack the ground when he walked. He had presented to the emergency department 1 month prior after he tripped on a sidewalk and struck his head, leaving him unconscious for a brief period of time. He also reported a 3-year history of burning pain in both feet, at times severe, accompanied by intermittent numbness.

He denied having difficulty chewing, swallowing, speaking, or shortness of breath. He did note urinary urgency and frequency, and in fact had experienced more than one episode of urinary incontinence recently. He had no bowel difficulties.

The patient had lost approximately 45 kg in weight over the previous year, which he stated was intentional due to dietary changes. He had undergone right shoulder surgery to repair a rotator cuff injury 3 years prior. He had undergone a remote appendectomy and had been involved in a motor vehicle collision at 15 years old that resulted in multiple fractures

and a shoulder injury. He was taking no medications and had no known allergies.

He was divorced and had two children. He had achieved a grade 12 education and worked as a commercial truck driver and transport coordinator. He reported drinking an average of two alcoholic beverages daily. He had stopped smoking 20 years previously. He denied any current or historical recreational drug use.

9.1.3 Family History

The patient's mother had a history of dementia, with onset in her early 60s. His mother was 1 of 11 children, and seven of them had suffered from dementia at unknown ages. The patient himself was the third eldest in a family of eight children, and none of his siblings were known to suffer from cognitive difficulties. The patient's children were unaffected. There was no other family history of neurological disease.

9.1.4 Examination

The patient's general medical examination was normal. He was alert and oriented but had difficulty conveying the specifics of his recent medical history. Language was intact with normal fluency, comprehension, repetition, and naming. Cognition was assessed with the Montreal Cognitive Assessment (MoCA) screening test, on which the patient scored 20/30, consistent with mild cognitive impairment. He struggled to copy a shape and was only able to name one of three animals. The patient also struggled with serial subtractions by seven and categorical abstraction. His delayed recall was one of five words.

On cranial nerve examination the patient had full extraocular movements without nystagmus and no ptosis. Facial motor and sensation were normal. His tongue was mildly atrophic with fasciculations. He had positive glabellar tap and bilateral palmomental reflexes. He had a positive grasp reflex.

Motor examination revealed decreased bulk in the spinati muscles as well as the thighs and lower legs bilaterally. Subtle fasciculations were evident in his shoulders and arms, with profuse fasciculations in

36

the legs bilaterally. Tone was normal in the upper extremities and increased in the lower extremities. Upper extremity power was Medical Research Council (MRC) grade 5 bilaterally. In the lower extremities he had reduced power with MRC grade 3/4+ (right/left) hip flexion, 4/4 hip abduction, 4/4 hip adduction, 3/5 knee extension, 3/5 knee flexion, 1/5 ankle dorsiflexion, and 2/5 ankle plantar flexion.

Deep tendon reflexes were 2+ in the upper extremities, 3+ at the knee, 2+ at the ankle, and symmetrical throughout. He had positive crossed adductor responses. His right plantar reflex was upgoing, while the left was downgoing.

Sensory examination was normal throughout the upper extremities. He had decreased pinprick and temperature sensation in a stocking distribution to the knees. Vibration sensation was absent and joint position sense was reduced in the right great toe, but normal on the left.

On coordination testing the patient had normal finger-to-nose and heel-to-shin tests. Gait was stable but notable for a significant right foot drop. Romberg sign was negative.

9.1.5 Special Studies

Magnetic resonance imaging (MRI) of the brain revealed nonspecific small vessel ischemic changes. Brain volume was well preserved for his age and there were no areas of focal atrophy. MRI of the spine was unremarkable. An FDG PET brain scan (Figure 9.1) revealed moderate hypometabolism in the frontal and anterior temporal lobes as well as the insular cortices and the anterior aspects of the cingulate gyri, in a pattern compatible with behavioral variant frontotemporal dementia (bvFTD).

Electromyographic studies revealed active denervation and fasciculations in the right leg and fasciculations in the right arm. Nerve conduction studies revealed no evidence of large fiber involvement. Initial studies did not strictly meet El Escorial criteria for motor neuron disease, although taken with the clinical exam were highly suggestive.

On serology the patient had a normal CBC, electrolytes, creatinine, liver enzymes, hemoglobin A1c, and urinalysis; vitamin B12 was supratherapeutic; TSH was borderline elevated; methylmalonic acid was normal; HIV, syphilis, and lyme serology were negative; lead and aluminum levels were normal; rheumatoid factor was negative; serum and urine protein electrophoresis were normal.

Neuropsychological testing was performed. On the amyotrophic lateral sclerosis (ALS) Cognitive Behavioral Screen he scored 14/20, consistent with severe impairment relative to healthy controls. He lost points on mental addition, tracking, and monitoring, and on initiation and retrieval tasks. On verbal skills testing, he had mildly impaired categorical fluency and severely impaired verbal abstract reasoning. Visuospatial skills, and attention and working memory were all generally intact. New learning and memory was impaired with verbal material (retention of 6/16 words over five learning trials) but intact with visuospatial material. On executive skills testing, he had semantic and language-related deficits including severely impaired verbal abstract reasoning, visuomotor tracking, and moderately impaired category fluency. Collectively, his neuropsychological profile was

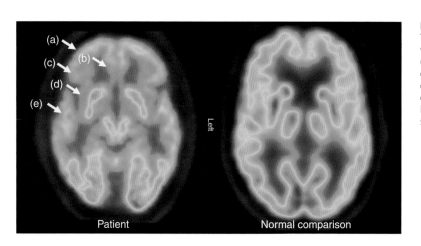

Figure 9.1 FDG PET imaging results. The patient (left) is shown in comparison with a normal study (right). Arrows indicate (a) frontal convexity, (b) anterior cingulate gyrus, (c) frontal operculum, (d) insular cortex, and (e) anterior temporal lobe. The changes are symmetric (but only one side indicated by arrows). The findings are suggestive of frontotemporal dementia.

suggestive of left hemisphere dysfunction suspicious for an emerging dementia.

Genetic testing confirmed *C9orf72* hexanucleotide expansion with 30 GGGGCC repeats (normal range 2–24).

9.1.6 Diagnosis

Electrophysiological studies were highly suggestive of motor neuron disease. In the context of the clinical exam and appearance of frontal lobe dysfunction, along with confirmation of *C9orf72* GGGGCC hexanucleotide repeat expansion, a diagnosis was made of ALS-FTD. The patient did not strictly meet International Consensus Criteria for probable bvFTD, given the absence of MRI findings consistent with bvFTD.[1] However, FDG PET results were strongly suggestive of the diagnosis of bvFTD and can be more sensitive in early disease. The presence of a known pathogenic genetic mutation for this phenotype provides a definitive diagnosis.

ALS-FTD was suspected when this patient first presented. The presence of upper and lower motor neuron weakness along with personality changes in a patient with a strong family history of dementia immediately raised suspicion for disease caused by autosomal dominantly inherited *C9orf72* hexanucleotide repeat expansion. Roughly 1 in 10 ALS patients carry *C9orf72* repeat expansion and FTD occurs in about half of these patients.[2] Given this frequency, *C9orf72* repeat expansion should be suspected in any ALS patient with a strong family history of ALS or FTD.

9.1.7 Follow-Up

The patient's motor function declined steadily. Six months after his initial presentation and subsequent diagnosis he began to urinate every 30 min, without sensation, and as a result he was regularly incontinent. Urodynamic studies led to a diagnosis of neurogenic overactive bladder and obstructive voiding. He had progressive loss of power along with muscle atrophy, increased fasciculations, and increased tone with spasticity. In addition to this he continued to suffer from severe burning in the lower extremity from a neuropathic pain that was long-standing and poorly responsive to treatment. Repeat electrophysiology studies 9 months after the patient first presented met El Escorial criteria for motor neuron disease.

The patient's driver's license was initially suspended due to concerns over cognition and motor strength. This was particularly concerning to the patient because his livelihood was based on driving. His behavior when discussing driving with his family and healthcare team was frequently aggressive and at times threatening. The patient challenged the driving test and regained his license for a brief period. He did not agree to stop driving until he had a low-speed collision with a post.

The patient's sisters began to note that he was gambling more frequently at the racetrack and losing significant amounts of money. He was also pursuing online scams that in the past he would not have considered according to family. He was unable to pay bills, which were being covered by his daughter. He was unconcerned by his inability to manage his finances. He had poor insight into his illness and was frequently in denial. He repeatedly refused home care support despite ongoing concern from his family for his safety.

Neuropsychological testing was repeated. He scored 13/20 on the ALS Cognitive Behavioral Screen and 110/144 on the Dementia Rating Scale, placing him in the severely impaired range. The assessment indicated declines in single-word recognition, category fluency, and phonemic fluency. He had a marked decline in confrontation naming with semantic paraphasic errors evident. He exhibited executive limitations including poor abstract reasoning, slow processing speed, and diminished sensitivity to punishment associated with decision-making impairment. Simple attention and working memory were intact, as was delayed recall for visuospatial information. His language decline had features of semantic variant primary progressive aphasia.

The patient was briefly admitted to hospital 1 year after his initial presentation with failure to thrive and frequent falls at home resulting in an ankle injury. On discharge he was transferred to a long-term care facility and a declaration of incapacity was completed. Shortly after transfer he was unable to reposition himself in bed and was requiring full lift transfers due to weakness. He was suffering from depressed mood that was not responsive to antidepressant medication. Nursing staff reported multiple episodes of aggression, verbal abuse, and at least one occasion of physical abuse. His behavior was a significant stress for his family, who were frequently forced to intervene to assist long-term care staff. The patient's family eventually decided to have him undergo stem cell treatment at an out-of-country private institution, against medical advice, resulting in no perceivable change in his condition.

9.2 Discussion

Amyotrophic lateral sclerosis (ALS) is a progressive neurodegenerative disease affecting both upper and lower motor neurons. FTD is characterized by progressive personality, behavioral, and/or language impairment due to frontal and temporal lobe cortical degeneration. The spectrum of FTD and motor neuron disease (MND) is characterized by overlapping clinical features, common underlying pathological mechanisms, genetics, and molecular mechanisms. It is now recognized that there is an inherited form of ALS with FTD (ALS-FTD) defined by a GGGGCC hexanucleotide repeat expansion in the chromosome 9 open reading frame 72 (C9orf72) gene.[3] Although no specific therapies exist for ALS or FTD, diagnosis has important implications for prognostication, care planning, and genetic counseling.

9.2.1 Epidemiology and Genetics

Up to 50% of patients with ALS experience cognitive dysfunction and about 5–10% have FTD.[4] Similarly, in one cohort study, about 15% of patients with FTD developed motor neuron dysfunction, although no population-based studies are available.[5]

Sporadic cases of FTD in association with ALS are also seen in conjunction with familial associations. The most common genetic cause of FTD-ALS is C9orf72 hexanucleotide repeat expansion.[6] Other rare mutations noted in cases of FTD-MND include valosin-containing protein (VCP), sequestosome 1 (SQSTM1), optineurin (OPTN), and ubiquilin 2 (UBQLN2).[7,8] C9orf72 repeat expansion is inherited in an autosomal dominant manner. It is estimated that 56% of familial FTD-ALS and 14% of sporadic FTD-ALS carry this repeat expansion.[9] The repeat tract length in unaffected individuals may vary between 5 and 10 and is usually <23. In patients with FTD-ALS, the tract is expanded to hundreds or thousands of repeats. Although it is unknown how many repeats are required to cause disease, the arbitrary cutoff for pathogenic repeats is set at 30, or 60 in some studies. The frequency is variable within population studies, with Caucasians reporting the highest carrier rate particularly in isolated populations such

as Finland (29%).[10,11] Age of onset is highly variable (27–85 years) with a mean of 58 years.[12] A slight male predominance (1.23:1) has been proposed for FTD-ALS cases with C9orf72 mutations. In familial cases of FTD-ALS, a younger age of onset was noted with progression of generations suggesting genetic anticipation.[12] The penetrance is currently unknown but thought to be incomplete. The cumulative age-dependent disease penetrance for C9orf72 heterozygous patients is 0% at age 35, 50% at age 58, and almost 100% at age 80.[10] The precise disease mechanism of this genetic lesion remains unknown. Three different mechanisms of disease have been proposed for the repeat expansion: loss of function of the gene, gain of protein toxicity due to expression of protein containing the expansion, and gain of RNA toxicity from the mutant RNA.[13]

9.2.2 Pathology

The phosphorylated form of TDP-43 is considered to be the underlying accumulating protein in susceptible areas in patients with FTD and ALS. In FTD, 40–50% of patients have TDP-43 inclusions whereas about 75–90% of ALS cases exhibit the same pathology.[8] There are four different pathological subtypes identified in FTD based on morphology and characteristics of inclusions (Type A–D). C9orf72 repeat expansion cases usually express Type B TDP-43 pathology.[14] A hierarchical pattern of infiltration of TDP-43 has been identified pathologically for both FTD and ALS with greatest overlap in Type B pathology. The pathology of FTD-ALS show loss of anterior horn and cranial nerve nuclei motor neurons with microglial activation in the corticospinal tracts in addition to TDP-43 deposition.[15] In addition, C9orf72 cases show presence of neuronal cytoplasmic inclusions and nuclear RNA foci that stain positive for ubiquitin and p62 but not for TDP-43[14] in extra motor regions such as hippocampal pyramidal neurons, and granular and molecular layers of the cerebellum.[16]

9.2.3 Clinical Features

The most common clinical phenotypes expressed with C9orf72 mutations is FTD, ALS, or a combination of both. FTD is currently recognized as the second most common etiology for dementia under age 65.[17] Three distinct clinical subtypes are currently recognized in FTD: bvFTD, semantic variant PPA, and nonfluent variant PPA. Individuals with

C9orf72-positive genetics demonstrate the bvFTD phenotype most frequently.[18] bvFTD with *C9orf72* expansion presents with the usual symptoms of disinhibition, apathy, loss of empathy, perseverative/compulsive behaviors, hyperorality, and impulsivity. In addition, psychotic symptoms are very common in *C9orf72* carriers including visual/auditory hallucinations and bizarre somatic delusions.[19] The presence of psychosis as a presenting feature makes the likelihood of having the *C9orf72* expansion more likely. The majority of patients lack insight at presentation. Primary progressive aphasias are an uncommon phenotype of *C9orf72* disease and in large series only a few cases have been described. There have also been reports of presentation with a phenotype including memory impairment and visuospatial dysfunction that resembles Alzheimer's disease. More than 50% of FTD patients who carry *C9orf72* expansions develop symptoms of motor neuron disease over the course of their disease progression.[15]

When patients with *C9orf72* expansion present with motor symptoms, they are often indistinguishable from classic ALS. *C9orf72* expansions are rarely causal to progressive muscular atrophy or primary lateral sclerosis.[20] ALS is a neurodegenerative disease characterized by a progressive decline in upper motor neurons and lower motor neurons. The most common form is limb onset (60–70%), followed by bulbar onset (speech and swallowing difficulties) in 30–40%.[21] In population-based studies about 10–15% of patients with ALS have met criteria for FTD. Progression is much more rapid and carries a worse prognosis in these cases. Clinically, patients with *C9orf72* repeat expansions have a higher incidence of bulbar onset ALS, cognitive impairment with early disease onset, and accelerated progression. Bulbar onset ALS and low education are proposed as risk factors for cognitive impairment.[22] Executive impairment is common even when criteria for FTD is not met and is present in 20–25% of cases with ALS. Patients with ALS demonstrated impairment in tasks such as assessing planning, monitoring of information, developing strategies, and mental set-shifting. Language-based dysfunction has also been noted in patients with motor neuron disease and independent of executive dysfunction. Difficulties in processing and recognizing facial emotions may partly account for emotional lability in bulbar onset ALS.[8] There is significant impairment of social cognition, theory of mind, and emotional processing.[23] Behavioral

symptoms can precede motor symptoms by 12 months, and although they do not change survival they do increase caregiver burden.

Other neurodegenerative disorders associated with *C9orf72* disease include parkinsonism, which has been also described in patients with *MAPT* and *GRN* mutations. In the absence of FTD or ALS, *C9orf72* expansions were present in patients with dementia with Lewy bodies, multiple system atrophy, and corticobasal syndrome.[24,25] Hyperkinetic movement disorders such as Huntington's disease have also shown *C9orf72* expansions in up to 2% of patients.[25]

The differential diagnosis for *C9orf72* repeat expansion-related FTD includes Alzheimer's disease, diffuse Lewy body dementia, Huntington's disease, and other forms of FTD. The differential diagnosis for patients presenting with ALS includes compressive (cervical) myeloradiculopathy, chronic inflammatory demyelinating polyradiculoneuropathy, multifocal motor, toxic or metabolic neuropathy and myopathies, and various forms of spinal muscular atrophy.[26]

9.2.4 Investigations

Assessment of a patient with possible FTD-ALS requires a thorough history from the patient and good collateral history from the caregiver or informant. A full neurological exam should be performed looking for signs of motor neuron disease, assessment of axial tone, presence of parkinsonism, cortical sensory tests, apraxia testing, and frontal release signs. Neuropsychological testing of *C9orf72*-positive patients has largely been retrospective in nature. Screening for behavioral symptoms can be done using ALS Cognitive Behavioral Screen, Frontal Systems Behavior Scale, and full-length neuropsychological testing evaluating the extent and profile of cognitive disturbance.[27] CSF biomarkers such as amyloid-β, total tau, phosphorylated tau, and their ratios may aid in distinguishing FTD from Alzheimer-type dementia if patients present with predominant memory complaints.[28] Electrophysiology studies may show widespread denervation and intact sensory responses consistent with a diagnosis of ALS, although reduced sensory responses have been noted. In the setting of normal electrophysiological studies, some patients with FTD may demonstrate fasciculations or other subtle motor neuron dysfunction. Neuroimaging, such as MRI, assists in ruling out etiologies such as vascular and structural abnormalities and allows for assessment of patterns of atrophy. Patients with *C9orf72* repeat expansion demonstrate atrophy of the frontal lobes with some involvement of the anterior temporal, parietal, and occipital lobes, and cerebellum and thalamus. SPECT and FDG PET studies have shown evidence of hypometabolism before atrophy is evident on MRI.[29] FDG PET studies have shown hypometabolic clusters in frontal and temporal cortex as neurobiological correlates of ALS with comorbid FTD.[30,31] When family history is suggestive of familial FTD, ALS, or FTD-ALS syndrome, a referral to a geneticist for genetic testing and counseling is recommended. In addition, an assessment for need of ancillary equipment or home occupational therapy assessment is recommended.

9.2.5 Management

The management of patients with comorbid FTD and motor neuron disease presents a unique set of challenges and no evidence-based guidelines are available. A multidisciplinary approach in treating ALS is well established and most helpful in dementia syndromes as well. Prognosis in FTD-ALS is poor with survival medians of 2–3 years from symptom onset.[32] Nonpharmacologic interventions include physical and occupational therapy, speech therapy, respiratory assistance, and a discussion regarding advance care planning. Home safety evaluations and implementation of communication devices are particularly helpful.

No specific therapies exist to manage abnormal behaviors. Intervention is recommended when behaviors are dangerous or too stressful for caregivers to manage. Although high-quality evidence is unavailable, selective serotonin reuptake inhibitors (SSRIs) are considered as the first-line treatment of behavioral symptoms. Venlafaxine is recommended when apathy is a prominent feature of the presentation.[8] Atypical antipsychotics are considered in patients with severe behavioral and psychological symptoms such as aggression, agitation, and psychosis. Although riluzole has clear indication in motor neuron disease, its role in the overlap of FTD-ALS is not well established. Other interventions, such as enteral feeding and non-invasive ventilation, although beneficial in ALS alone have no direct evidence in FTD-ALS.[33] Compliance with such intervention may also be problematic as behavioral symptoms progress over the course of the disease.

Caregiver burden is often significant, secondary to multiple behavioral problems, and psychosocial support and education is recommended to reduce stress. In later stages, regular respite for caregivers is essential and placement in a supervised living environment may be necessary.

9.2.6 Future Directions

Much about *C9orf72* repeat expansion is not well delineated including minimum pathogenic length of repeat expansion, mechanisms of neurodegeneration, biomarkers of disease onset and progression, guidelines for genetic counseling, and drug candidates for pilot studies. Recent trials in motor neuron disease are looking at genetics of familial and sporadic ALS, imaging and biomarkers in ALS, and mechanisms of neuroinflammation in ALS. In the future, we will need reliable data about disease penetrance of *C9orf72* repeat expansion for purposes of genetic counseling. Further in vivo and in vitro models to answer questions regarding neurodegenerative mechanisms and to formulate therapeutic targets will be essential. Validation of cognitive questionnaires in motor neuron disease and screening for motor neuron dysfunction in dementia will be helpful for diagnostic and prognostication purposes. Given the clinical heterogeneity and variability in presentation, diagnosis, prognostication, and therapeutics will be challenging for this spectrum of disorders.

References

1. Rascovsky K, Hodges JR, Knopman D, et al. Sensitivity of revised diagnostic criteria for the behavioural variant of frontotemporal dementia. *Brain*. 2011;134(Pt 9): 2456–2477. doi:10.1093/brain/awr179.

2. Byrne S, Elamin M, Bede P, et al. Cognitive and clinical characteristics of patients with amyotrophic lateral sclerosis carrying a C9orf72 repeat expansion: a population-based cohort study. *Lancet Neurol*. 2012;11(3):232–240. doi:10.1016/S1474-4422(12) 70014-5.

3. Morita M, Al-Chalabi A, Andersen PM, et al. A locus on chromosome 9p confers susceptibility to ALS and frontotemporal dementia. *Neurology*. 2006;66(6):839–844. doi:10.1212/01. wnl.0000200048.53766.b4.

4. Goldstein LH, Abrahams S. Changes in cognition and

behaviour in amyotrophic lateral sclerosis: nature of impairment and implications for assessment. *Lancet Neurol.* 2013;12 (4):368–380. doi:10.1016/S1474-4422(13)70026-7.

5. Lomen-Hoerth C, Anderson T, Miller B. The overlap of amyotrophic lateral sclerosis and frontotemporal dementia. *Neurology.* 2002;59(7):1077–1079.

6. Renton AE, Majounie E, Waite A, et al. A hexanucleotide repeat expansion in C9ORF72 is the cause of chromosome 9p21-linked ALS-FTD. *Neuron.* 2011;72 (2):257–268. doi:10.1016/j. neuron.2011.09.010.

7. Al-Chalabi A, Hardiman O. The epidemiology of ALS: a conspiracy of genes, environment and time. *Nat Rev Neurol.* 2013;9 (11):617–628. doi:10.1038/ nrneurol.2013.203.

8. Burrell JR, Halliday GM, Kril JJ, et al. The frontotemporal dementia-motor neuron disease continuum. *Lancet.* 2016;388 (10047):919–931. doi:10.1016/ S0140-6736(16)00737-6.

9. van der Zee J, Gijselinck I, Dillen L, et al. A pan-European study of the C9orf72 repeat associated with FTLD: geographic prevalence, genomic instability, and intermediate repeats. *Hum Mutat.* 2013;34(2):363–373. doi:10.1002/ humu.22244.

10. Majounie E, Renton AE, Mok K, et al. Frequency of the C9orf72 hexanucleotide repeat expansion in patients with amyotrophic lateral sclerosis and frontotemporal dementia: a cross-sectional study. *Lancet Neurol.* 2012;11(4):323–330. doi:10.1016/ S1474-4422(12)70043-1.

11. Mok K, Traynor BJ, Schymick J, et al. Chromosome 9 ALS and FTD locus is probably derived from a single founder. *Neurobiol Aging.* 2012;33(1): 209.e3-8. doi:10.1016/j. neurobiolaging.2011.08.005.

12. Boeve BF, Boylan KB, Graff-Radford NR, et al. Characterization of frontotemporal dementia and/or amyotrophic lateral sclerosis associated with the GGGGCC repeat expansion in C9ORF72. *Brain.* 2012;135(Pt 3):765–783. doi:10.1093/brain/aws004.

13. Yokoyama JS, Sirkis DW, Miller BL. C9ORF72 hexanucleotide repeats in behavioral and motor neuron disease: clinical heterogeneity and pathological diversity. *Am J Neurodegener Dis.* 2014;3(1):1–18.

14. Mackenzie IR, Frick P, Neumann M. The neuropathology associated with repeat expansions in the C9ORF72 gene. *Acta Neuropathol.* 2014;127(3):347–357. doi:10.1007/ s00401-013-1232-4.

15. Snowden JS, Rollinson S, Thompson JC, et al. Distinct clinical and pathological characteristics of frontotemporal dementia associated with C9ORF72 mutations. *Brain.* 2012;135(Pt 3):693–708. doi:10.1093/brain/awr355.

16. Cooper-Knock J, Hewitt C, Highley JR, et al. Clinico-pathological features in amyotrophic lateral sclerosis with expansions in C9ORF72. *Brain.* 2012;135(Pt 3): 751–764. doi:10.1093/brain/ awr365.

17. Knopman DS, Petersen RC, Edland SD, Cha RH, Rocca WA. The incidence of frontotemporal lobar degeneration in Rochester, Minnesota, 1990 through 1994. *Neurology.* 2004;62(3):506–508.

18. Cooper-Knock J, Shaw PJ, Kirby J. The widening spectrum of C9ORF72-related disease; genotype/phenotype correlations and potential modifiers of clinical phenotype. *Acta Neuropathol.* 2014;127(3):333–345. doi:10.1007/ s00401-014-1251-9.

19. Devenney E, Hornberger M, Irish M, et al. Frontotemporal dementia

associated with the C9ORF72 mutation: a unique clinical profile. *JAMA Neurol.* 2014;71 (3):331–339. doi:10.1001/ jamaneurol.2013.6002.

20. van Rheenen W, van Blitterswijk M, Huisman MH, et al. Hexanucleotide repeat expansions in C9ORF72 in the spectrum of motor neuron diseases. *Neurology.* 2012;79(9):878–882. doi:10.1212/ WNL.0b013e3182661d14.

21. Cruts M, Gijselinck I, Van Langenhove T, van der Zee J, Van Broeckhoven C. Current insights into the C9orf72 repeat expansion diseases of the FTLD/ALS spectrum. *Trends Neurosci.* 2013;36(8):450–459. doi:10.1016/j. tins.2013.04.010.

22. Chio A, Borghero G, Restagno G, et al. Clinical characteristics of patients with familial amyotrophic lateral sclerosis carrying the pathogenic GGGGCC hexanucleotide repeat expansion of C9ORF72. *Brain.* 2012;135(Pt 3):784–793. doi:10.1093/brain/ awr366.

23. Girardi A, Macpherson SE, Abrahams S. Deficits in emotional and social cognition in amyotrophic lateral sclerosis. *Neuropsychology.* 2011;25 (1):53–65. doi:10.1037/a0020357.

24. Lindquist SG, Duno M, Batbayli M, et al. Corticobasal and ataxia syndromes widen the spectrum of C9ORF72 hexanucleotide expansion disease. *Clin Genet.* 2013;83(3):279–283. doi:10.1111/ j.1399-0004.2012.01903.x.

25. Liu Y, Yu JT, Zong Y, Zhou J, Tan L. C9ORF72 mutations in neurodegenerative diseases. *Mol Neurobiol.* 2014;49(1), 386–398. doi:10.1007/s12035-013-8528-1.

26. Cruts M, Engelborghs S, van der Zee J, Van Broeckhoven C. C9orf72-related amyotrophic lateral sclerosis and frontotemporal dementia. In: Pagon, RA, Adam MP, Ardinger

HH, et al., eds. *GeneReviews(R)*. Seattle, WA: University of Washington; 1993.

27. Woolley SC, York MK, Moore DH, et al. Detecting frontotemporal dysfunction in ALS: utility of the ALS Cognitive Behavioral Screen (ALS-CBS). *Amyotroph Lateral Scler*. 2010;11 (3):303–311. doi:10.3109/ 17482961003727954.

28. Skillback T, Farahmand BY, Rosen C, et al. Cerebrospinal fluid tau and amyloid-beta1–42 in patients with dementia. *Brain*. 2015;138(Pt 9):2716–2731. doi:10.1093/brain/awv181.

29. Sha SJ, Takada LT, Rankin KP, et al. Frontotemporal dementia due to C9ORF72 mutations: clinical and imaging features. *Neurology*. 2012;79 (10):1002–1011. doi:10.1212/ WNL.0b013e318268452e.

30. Canosa A, Pagani M, Cistaro A, et al. 18F-FDG-PET correlates of cognitive impairment in ALS. *Neurology*. 2016;86(1):44–49. doi:10.1212/ WNL.0000000000002242.

31. Lomen-Hoerth C. Clinical phenomenology and neuroimaging correlates in ALS-FTD. *J Mol Neurosci*. 2011;45

(3):656–662. doi:10.1007/s12031-011-9636-x.

32. Coon EA, Sorenson EJ, Whitwell JL, Knopman DS, Josephs KA. Predicting survival in frontotemporal dementia with motor neuron disease. *Neurology*. 2011;76(22):1886–1893. doi:10.1212/ WNL.0b013e31821d767b.

33. Rohrer JD, Isaacs AM, Mizielinska S, et al. C9orf72 expansions in frontotemporal dementia and amyotrophic lateral sclerosis. *Lancet Neurol*. 2015;14 (3):291–301. doi:10.1016/S1474-4422(14)70233-9.

A Woman with Progressive Episodic Memory Loss and Personality Change

Rodrigo A. Santibanez, Ian R. A. Mackenzie, and Ging-Yuek R. Hsiung

10.1 Case History

A 62-year-old right-handed lady presented at initial consultation with an 18 months history of slowly progressive short-term memory problems and personality change. She denied having any problems herself, suggesting some lack of insight. However, the collateral history obtained from her daughter made it clear that she had problems with progressive worsening of her short-term memory in the past 18 months, severe enough to be of concern in the last year. She reported that she had a poor episodic memory for conversations and recent events. As an example, her daughter gave examples that the patient was frequently unable to remember previous conversations. Also, she mentioned that she was prone to forget the discussed topic in the middle of conversations.

She did not have difficulties remembering proper nouns or recognizing people. Her semantic memory and long-term memory seemed to be well preserved, and her recall of past events was accurate. Her daughter mentioned that her organizational abilities declined compared to her previous skills, for example, she was having problems keeping track of her credit card and finances. Regarding her language, her daughter noted occasional naming problems. Her language output was normal, as well as her grammar. No paraphasias were noted. Her speech was also normal. Her daughter described her visuospatial skills and topographic orientation as being good.

From the psychobehavioral standpoint, her daughter reported that her personality had changed. She used to be a short-tempered and anxious person, but she became calmer and much more easy going. On the other hand, she also showed some increased impulsive behavior, such as shouting at cashiers when she had problems paying for items when shopping. Also, she was spending in excess and giving away her money indiscriminately; as an example, once she bought seven leather jackets in a day, and she gave money to a family member with addiction problems. No other behavioral issues were noted, and her mood was generally described as upbeat and stable. There were no hallucinations. She had no obsessive behaviors. Her

sleeping pattern was fine, with no evidence of REM sleep behavior disorder or any other parasomnia, but she has a long history of benzodiazepine use. Her appetite was normal with no change in her eating preferences. There were no motor issues, no tremor, no falls.

Functionally, she was independent with her basic activities of daily living. However, she had impairment in some of her instrumental activities. As an example, she was having problems with her finances.

10.2 Past Medical History

Her past medical history was notable for diabetes mellitus type 2 and hypothyroidism for over 5 years. She was on metformin 500 mg two times a day, pravastatin 20 mg/day, spironolactone 50 mg/day, levothyroxine 0.075 mg/day, and oxazepam 15–30 mg every night at bedtime for sleep, for a long time, due to insomnia starting in her 40s.

On review of her risk factors for dementia, it was noted that she had a 50 pack-year history of smoking. Additionally, she was a heavy drinker in her 30s, when she also had problems with depression that required hospitalization and antidepressant treatments. At the time of the initial consultation, she was still drinking, but only a glass of wine occasionally. She had no significant head injuries. There were no stroke-like episodes or other neurological symptoms.

10.3 Family History

Her mother died at 61 from heart attack and had no cognitive problems at the time. Her father also died at 84 from heart problems and was mentally alert. There is no information on the extended family history.

The patient was the 12th born of 15 children. Two died in childbirth. One sister died at 32 from brain aneurysm. From the remaining siblings, two brothers and one sister developed early-onset dementia in their late 50s, passing away in their early 60s. No autopsies were performed. Medical records were only available on one family member, and that was compatible with probable Alzheimer's dementia.

10.4 Social History

The patient was born in the province of Manitoba with French ancestry on the maternal side and Polish ancestry on the father's side. She had a grade six education and worked as a clerk and waitress in the past. She was married for the third time and her husband was suffering from several chronic medical problems that were limiting his mobility and independence. She had a daughter and a son.

10.5 Clinical Examination

Her general physical examination was normal. Her blood pressure was 120/70, with a regular pulse of 76. She had no cranial or carotid bruits. Breath sounds were clear and heart sounds were normal. Abdomen was soft, lax with no organomegaly. Her peripheral pulses were intact. She had no lower limb edema.

She was alert and mostly cooperative during examination and not under stress, but occasionally irritable. She was well dressed and in good hygiene. She did not exhibit any abnormal behavior, stereotypic or utilization behavior. Her speech was normal.

On cognitive assessment, she scored 24/30 on MMSE and 77/100 on 3MS. She lost points on mental reversal, and temporal and spatial orientation from the MMSE, but was able to remember three words. On the 3MS she lost further points on naming four-legged animals, describing similarities. She also made mistakes scoring 2/3 on the three-stage command.

On more detailed cognitive assessment, her spontaneous language and verbal output was normal with no lexical retrieval difficulties, paraphasias, or dysarthria. Her phonemic fluency was impaired, naming only four words beginning with letter S in 1 min. Her visual confrontation naming was also impaired, managing to name three out of six objects with a slight improvement after lexical cues. Her semantic knowledge about those objects was preserved.

In her logical memory testing, there was evidence of short-term memory impairment noted on her paragraph-free recall of specific details, but the concept was retained.

Her executive functioning also demonstrated impairment on testing, with problems on abstractions and describing similarities. She completed the three-step Luria Sequence easily.

Her visuospatial functioning was abnormal. While her free clock drawing was intact, she made a number of errors copying a 3D cube. On a task of visuospatial problem solving, she scored 5/6 on square fitting.

Cranial nerves: Pupils were equal and reactive. Saccades and smooth pursuit were normal. She had no facial weakness or asymmetry. Palatal function, gag, and tongue movements were normal.

Motor: There was no drift on her outstretched upper limbs. Tone, power and bulk were normal. No other motor abnormalities were noted. Deep tendon reflexes were 2 in the upper and lower extremities. Plantar responses were both flexor. There was no parkinsonism and no abnormal movements at her initial assessment.

Sensory: The primary modalities of sensation were normal in the upper and lower extremities.

Coordination: Finger-to-nose and heel-to-shin responses were accurate. Tandem balance and her speed of movements were normal.

10.6 Additional Investigations

Blood work including blood count, liver function, electrolytes, renal function, Ca, thyroid function, folate, and B12 were in the normal range.

CT head scan showed no evidence of any structural lesions. However, it did show early atrophy, more prominent in the frontotemporal sulci compared to the posterior parietal region.

MRI showed no evidence of any structural lesions. However, it showed generalized atrophy with increased cerebral sulci, greater than expected for her age. The atrophy was more pronounced in the temporal lobes, while hippocampus appeared normal.

10.7 Neuroimaging

10.7.1 Clinical Diagnosis

The patient was initially diagnosed as an atypical presentation of Alzheimer's disease.

10.7.2 Clinical Course

On the following 3 years, the patient developed problems in multiple cognitive domains, with a prominent short-term memory impairment, lexical retrieval difficulties, and spatial disorientation on repeated testing. She continued to have executive dysfunction and visuospatial abnormalities. Later on, she developed face recognition problems, with no apparent semantic memory issues. Her behavior continued to show impulsivity and carelessness, but the decline in these aspects was significantly less prominent than in her memory and orientation. A mild hyperorality was also noted, with increased appetite. No other psychobehavioral problems emerged. Her cognitive scores showed a noticeable and fast decline, especially after the second year. Three years after the initial assessment, she scored 4/30 on MMSE and 11/100 on 3MS.

Follow-up neurological examination did not show significant changes from the first visit. The patient did not develop any cranial nerve abnormalities, muscular weakness, parkinsonism, or abnormal movements.

Initially, there was a slight improvement after a trial of donepezil, but later she had to discontinue the medication due to gastrointestinal side effects after 6 months. Then, she was switched to rivastigmine, but no improvement in her cognition was noted. Later on, she was put on memantine, with no obvious effect.

She remained functionally stable for 2 years when she was still able to live by herself, but afterward, her decline accelerated and she had to move to a care home for safety by year 3.

10.7.3 Final Impression

Her clinical diagnosis was an atypical presentation of Alzheimer's disease. However, a frontotemporal dementia was not completely ruled out because of some of her atypical clinical manifestation, such as rapid progression and prominent executive dysfunction early in the course with some behavioral changes.

10.7.4 Further Follow-Up

By the fifth year, she was completely dependent and required full-time assistance in a care facility. After she died of pneumonia, an autopsy was performed.

10.7.5 Neuropathology Findings

10.7.5.1 Gross Description

The brain weighed 884 g in the fresh state. Diffuse cerebral atrophy was noted with some sparing of the pre- and post-central gyrus. Serial coronal sections through the cerebral hemispheres confirmed a severe degree of cerebral atrophy with marked symmetric dilatation of the ventricular system. The atrophy was somewhat more pronounced in the frontal and temporal regions but also affected the parietal lobes. There was a moderate atrophy of the head of the caudate nucleus.

10.7.5.2 Microscopic Examination

Sections of cerebral neocortex showed loss of neurons with reactive changes and degeneration of the subcortical white matter that was severe in the frontal and temporal lobes but relatively mild in the parietal region. The neuronal population of the hippocampus was relatively intact. Bielschowsky silver stain failed to demonstrate any senile plaques and classical flame-shaped neurofibrillary tangles were rare (Figure 10.1a). However, there are abundant tau-immunoreactive neuronal and glial inclusions throughout the hippocampus, cerebral cortex, and a number of subcortical gray matter structures (Figure 10.1b). In the neocortex and hippocampus, neuronal inclusions predominate and include thin perinuclear crescents and annular rings as well as multiple small round or oval cytoplasmic bodies (Figure 10.2a). An even larger number of neurons demonstrate diffuse cytoplasmic tau immunoreactivity. The cortical neuropil also contains abundant small tau-immunoreactive dot- and thread-like processes (Figure 10.2b). In subcortical regions, chronic degenerative changes and tau pathology are most abundant in the basal ganglia, thalamus, substantia nigra, and periaqueductal gray matter (Figure 10.3). The most common glial inclusions appear as clusters of coarse granules adjacent to glial nuclei that decorate but do not completely fill the cell processes.

There were no Pick bodies, Lewy bodies, or TDP-43 immunoreactive inclusions.

Overall, the pathology in this case is similar to what has previously been described as "multiple system tauopathy with dementia." This terminology has been used for both sporadic cases with an FTD phenotype and some families found to harbor MAPT mutations.[1]

Final neuropathological diagnosis: Multiple system tauopathy with dementia.

10.7.6 Genetic Testing

Because of the extensive tau pathology found in this case, the patient's DNA was sent for research screening for tau mutation, and a P301L mutation was identified in the *MAPT* gene.

10.8 Discussion

Since the discovery of mutations in the microtubule-associated protein tau gene (*MAPT* on Chr17.q21.1) as a cause of frontotemporal dementia with parkinsonism linked to chromosome 17 (FTDP-17),[2] it has been shown that the clinical syndrome with MAPT mutations is highly heterogeneous, which can include behavioral variant frontotemporal dementia,

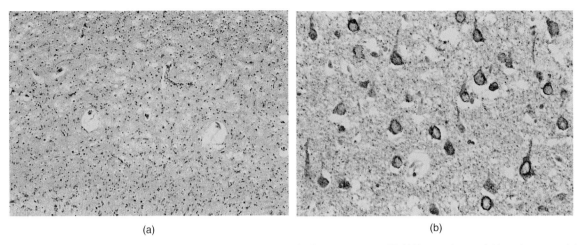

Figure 10.1 (a) Temporal cortex (in Bielschowsky stain ×10). No senile plaques, very rare NFT. (b) Temporal cortex (with tau immunostaining ×40). Numerous tau+ NFT, pre-tangles in neurons and granular dots in neuropil.

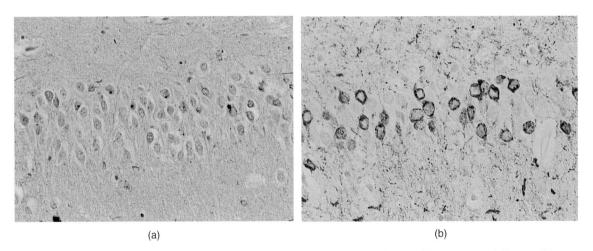

Figure 10.2 (a) Hippocampus (HC Biel ×40) shows only rare inclusions with Bielschowsky stain. (b) Hippocampus (HC tau ×40) demonstrating abundant tau+ pre-tangles.

nonfluent/agrammatic primary progressive aphasia, late-onset parkinsonism that overlaps with progressive supranuclear palsy and corticobasal syndrome, as well as memory disorders that mimics Alzheimer's disease.[3] While the degree of focal atrophy in the frontal and temporal regions can be variable depending on the clinical phenotype, there is often extensive neuronal loss, gliosis, and spongiosis in the superficial cortical layers found in routine microscopic staining in neuropathological studies. Immunohistochemical studies invariably show pathologic accumulation of hyperphosphorylated tau protein in all individuals with *MAPT* mutations, similar to our current case.[4,5]

Of all the mutations in *MAPT* reported to date, the most frequently observed changes are a C to T substitution corresponding to P301L in exon 10, as in our case.[6] Almost all *MAPT* mutations are heterozygous and segregated as dominant mutations within families. Based on the properties of the nucleotide changes, it is predicted that a stem-loop RNA structure spanning the splice donor site of intron 10 would be involved in regulation of exon 10 alternative splicing. It is hypothesized that the intronic mutations destabilized the stem-loop, altering the splicing machinery to favor the splicing-in of exon 10 and resulting in an increase in 4-repeat tau isoform level.[2,7]

47

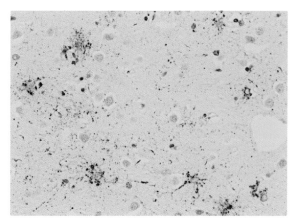

Figure 10.3 Basal ganglia (with tau immunostaining ×40) demonstrating numerous glial inclusions with beaded appearance.

The natural history of FTD is also highly variable depending on the clinical phenotype. Those with behavioral variant FTD tend to have a faster rate of decline and a shorter survival than those with language deficits initially. Those semantic dementia or non-fluent progressive aphasia tend to have longer survival, similar to AD.[8] Sudden and unexplained deaths are also more common in FTD.[9] In our case,

the rate of decline was faster than expected, which raised the suspicion that it was not a typical AD presentation. However, without biomarkers, it is difficult to be certain of the underlying pathology due to the overlapping symptomatology of the dementia syndromes. Current research efforts in defining biomarkers will be invaluable when disease-modifying therapies specific to the underlying pathology become available.

10.9 Take-Home Message

It is prudent to be vigilant of the heterogeneous presentation of MAPT-associated dementia and consider screening for genetic mutations in patients with a family history of autosomal dominant early-onset dementia.

Acknowledgments

Dr. Hsiung is supported by a Canadian Institute of Health Research Clinical Genetics Investigatorship award and the Ralph Fisher and Alzheimer Society of British Columbia Professorship.

References

1. Bigio EH, Lipton AM, Yen SH, et al. Frontal lobe dementia with novel tauopathy: sporadic multiple system tauopathy with dementia. *J Neuropathol Exp Neurol.* 2001;60(4):328–341.

2. Hutton M, Lendon CL, Rizzu P, et al. Association of missense and 5′-splice-site mutations in tau with the inherited dementia FTDP-17. *Nature.* 1998;393(6686):702–705.

3. Kertesz A. Pick's complex and FTDP-17. *Mov Disord.* 2003;18 (Suppl 6):S57–S62.

4. Pickering-Brown SM, Richardson AM, Snowden JS, et al. Inherited frontotemporal dementia in nine British families associated with intronic mutations in the tau gene. *Brain.* 2002;125(Pt 4):732–751.

5. Spillantini MG, Goedert M, Crowther RA, et al. Familial multiple system tauopathy with presenile dementia: a disease with abundant neuronal and glial tau filaments. *Proc Natl Acad Sci USA.* 1997;94(8):4113–4118.

6. Rademakers R, Cruts M, van Broeckhoven C. The role of tau (MAPT) in frontotemporal dementia and related tauopathies. *Hum Mutat.* 2004;24 (4):277–295.

7. Spillantini MG, Murrell JR, Goedert M, et al. Mutation in the tau gene in familial multiple system tauopathy with presenile dementia. *Proc Natl Acad Sci USA.* 1998;95 (13):7737–7741.

8. Roberson ED, Hesse JH, Rose KD, et al. Frontotemporal dementia progresses to death faster than Alzheimer disease. *Neurology.* 2005;65(5):719–725.

9. Pasquier F, Richard F, Lebert F. Natural history of frontotemporal dementia: comparison with Alzheimer's disease. *Dement Geriatr Cogn Disord.* 2004;17 (4):253–257.

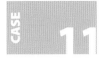

Left-Handed Man with Memory Complaints

Donnabelle Chu, Ian R. A. Mackenzie, and Ging-Yuek R. Hsiung

11.1 Case History

A 69-year old, left-handed man presented at initial consultation with a history of difficulty with short-term recall for 18 months. There were neither obvious behavioral changes nor changes in long-term memory. He also denied any difficulty with lexical retrieval. There was no difficulty in comprehension and no topographic disorientation. He would occasionally feel down, but it seemed to be appropriate to the situation with no sustained depression. On collateral history from his wife, she noted that the cognitive symptoms began about 3 years prior. This was described as gradually progressive memory loss initially having difficulty in recalling recent events, and then subsequently needing written cues or reminders for appointments. An example of this was he could not recall who they had dinner with from several nights prior. Another would be he would tend to forget that they had just eaten recently and could not recall what they ate.

His wife also noted some lexical retrieval problems with him and he was less sure of directions when driving. There was no note of any personality or behavioral changes and he still had a good sense of humor. No hallucinations or language problems were noted. He had nocturia and had difficulty in going back to sleep afterward, but there were no nightmares or excessive movements during sleep. Functionally, he was independent on activities of daily living and able to do household chores such as cleaning the windows. He can care for himself and is aware of the financial situation. He still was able to go shopping and prepare his meal, though at times somewhat forgetful.

From his neurologic review, his gait was noted to be slightly slower, but his balance remained good and still managed to climb a ladder without any concern. There were no involuntary movements noted, nor any visual changes or diplopia. There was no difficulty with chewing, swallowing, or speech, and no problems with fine motor control. He would only occasionally have mild headaches occurring once a week and was mostly stress related.

11.2 Past Medical History

He was diagnosed with rheumatic fever at age 54 but no other details were available. There were no reports of chest pain or palpitations. He was prone to indigestion but otherwise no gastrointestinal symptoms. He was recently diagnosed to have prostate cancer with an elevated PSA level requiring further management. He had no regular medication and had no known allergies.

On review of his risk factors for dementia, it was noted that he had chronic use of alcohol daily (2–3 oz) but no history of smoking. There have not been any sustained symptoms of depression, though it was noted that his wife felt there is some dysphoria at times. There was no history of head injury.

11.3 Family History

There was a strong history of dementia over at least three generations on his maternal side. Most prominent was that of his brother, who was evaluated at age 57 and was diagnosed with Alzheimer's dementia. He died at age 62 with an autopsy reporting changes consistent with dementia of the Alzheimer-type (reported in 1990s), although his history also mentioned significant executive dysfunction and personality change. His mother died at age 76 with dementia; however no autopsy was done. His maternal grandmother had late onset dementia with symptom onset at 88. She was provisionally diagnosed with "chronic brain syndrome due to senile brain disease," with psychotic reaction and was 96 years old at the time of death.

He was the eldest of three siblings. His younger brother died at age 62 (as mentioned above) and one younger sister who was healthy with no memory or cognitive problem. His father died at age 94 after a fall with no reported cases of dementia from his paternal family.

11.4 Social History

The patient was born in Vancouver, BC, and completed high school. He was of English ancestry both from his paternal and maternal side. He worked as a pharmaceutical salesman for 13 years and retired at the age of 61 with no problems with work at that time. He was married for 43 years and had two daughters and two grandchildren.

11.5 Initial Clinical Examination

The patient was fully cooperative during the examination, blood pressure was 150/70 mmHg and pulse rate of 72, with occasional ectopy. His general examination was notable for the absence of cranial or carotid bruits. He had a grade II/VI systolic murmur at the apex, radiating to the base. Abdominal examination was unremarkable. Skin and joints were also normal.

On cognitive assessment, he had a score of 21/30 on Mini-Mental State Examination (MMSE) and 67/100 on 3MS. On more detailed testing, he was noted to be significantly temporally disoriented while spatially oriented. He encoded test objects readily. At 5 min, he recalled 1/5 objects spontaneously, 2/5 with categorical cueing, and 3/5 with forced choices. There were some syntax errors noted when reading out a paragraph aloud. There was also a significant loss of concept in detail on this memory task.

On test of language, he was fluent in his ability to generate a word list to semantic category (11 four-legged animals in 30 s). Body part naming was normal. He named 8/10 items visually presented, improving with minimal cueing to nine. He had some restriction in his ability to abstract similarities. He did have difficulty with hand length on the clock drawing, suggesting some degree of visuospatial deficits.

He did perform the Luria hand sequences normally. There were some difficulties on tests of mental control, particularly in serial 7s (2/5) and other mental calculations. There were no frontal release reflexes.

Cranial nerves: Visual fields were full to confrontation. Discs were visualized and were normal. Extraocular movements were normal. No facial weakness with palatal function and speech normal.

Motor: There were no abnormalities in his upper and lower extremities.

Reflexes: DTRs were 2+ and symmetric bilaterally and both plantar responses were flexor.

Sensory: There were no abnormalities to the primary modalities tested.

Coordination: Finger-to-nose and heel-to-shin responses were accurate. His gait appeared to be slightly slow, but steady.

11.6 Additional Investigations

Blood works such as CBC, B12, folate, TSH, RPR, and FTA-ABS were all within normal range.

A computed tomography (CT) scan of the head with contrast showed mild degree of diffuse cortical tissue loss, no focal lesion seen.

Magnetic resonance imaging (MRI) of the brain showed bilateral temporal lobe atrophy with marked prominence of both Sylvian fissures. There was less marked atrophy with the frontal and parietal lobes. Several nonspecific high-signal foci within the left corona radiata and right centrum semiovale were also noted as well as a left temporal arachnoid cyst.

11.7 Clinical Diagnosis

The patient was initially diagnosed with mild dementia most consistent with Alzheimer's disease.

11.8 Clinical Course

The patient was serially followed and was noted to have progression of his short-term memory problem. In a 17-month period, he was unable to remember any appointments and recent events. He was also noted to have organizational difficulties and unable to complete household tasks. He was also noted to have topographic disorientation and had to stop driving. His mood became apathetic with less interests in any social activities, and he would have occasional delusions or confusion that his deceased parents were still alive. On testing, his MMSE and 3MS had no significant change with 22/30 on MMSE (prior 22/30) and 69/100 on 3MS (prior 67/100). There was clear executive dysfunction with difficulty on mental control and divided attention. He had impairment in retrieval and some perseverative behaviors were observed. Generative naming was reduced but verbal fluency remained good. Follow-up elemental neurological examination did not show any significant changes with only slight difficulty in tandem gait. He was started on donepezil 5 mg, which was later on increased to 10 mg; however, due to increased urinary frequency with no prominent cognitive improvement, the intake of donepezil was maintained on 5 mg daily.

On his subsequent follow-up (32 months after initial assessment), he had declined further, with an MMSE of 19/30 and 3MS of 59/100. His short-term and long-term memory had worsened, with occasions of getting lost. He was perseverative about helping out around the house, but could really not do anything unless supervised. He did not initiate any activity on his own, and needed help with dressing and personal hygiene. No specific behavioral changes were noted nor hallucinations, but he would need to be reminded on personal hygiene. He started to attend Adult Day Care three times a week for 6 h/day. He was maintained on donepezil 5 mg daily.

He expired 7 years after initial assessment at age 76, and an autopsy was subsequently performed.

11.9 Final Clinical Impression

Insidious onset, progressive dementia, probable Alzheimer's disease with significant memory loss. However, because of the strong family history and an atypical course, genetic cause of dementia was pursued.

11.10 Neuropathology Findings

11.10.1 Gross Description

The brain weighed 947 g in fresh state. There was severe cerebral atrophy with the left cerebral hemisphere affected more than the right. The frontal and temporal lobes were most severely involved; however, the parietal and occipital regions are also abnormal. No focal lesions were identified with minimal atherosclerosis of the major intracranial vessels. Serial coronal sections through the cerebral hemispheres confirmed severe atrophy, which dramatically affected the left hemisphere. There was marked atrophy of the striatum with more modest involvement of the lentiform nucleus and thalamus. Both hippocampi were small as well as the midbrain with loss of pigmentation of the substantia nigra.

11.11 Microscopic Examination

Sections of the frontal and temporal neocortex showed severe neuronal loss and reactive gliosis. Ubiquitin and TDP-43 immunohistochemistry demonstrated numerous short neurites, round and arcuate neuronal cytoplasmic inclusions, and rare lentiform neuronal intranuclear inclusions within

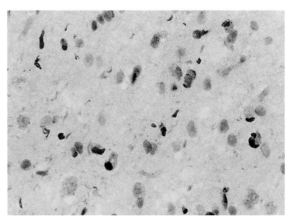

Figure 11.1 Layer 2 of the frontal neocortex with TDP-43 immunohistochemistry (60× magnification).

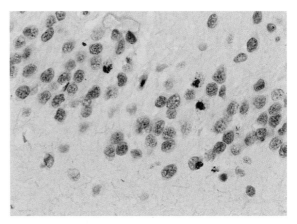

Figure 11.2 Hippocampal dentate layer with TDP-43 immunohistochemistry (60× magnification).

the superficial layers of the neocortex (Figure 11.1). Ubiquitin- and TDP-43-immunoreactive neuronal cytoplasmic inclusions were also present within the dentate granule layer of the hippocampus (Figure 11.2), and there was near complete loss of pyramidal neurons from CA1 and subiculum, consistent with hippocampal sclerosis (Figure 11.3). Moderate numbers of diffuse senile plaques were demonstrated with Bielschowsky silver method; however, neuritic senile plaques were sparse and tau-immunoreactive neurofibrillary tangles and neuropil threads were restricted to the entorhinal and transentorhinal cortex (Braak stage II). No other tau or alpha-synuclein-positive pathological changes were identified. There was severe chronic degeneration of

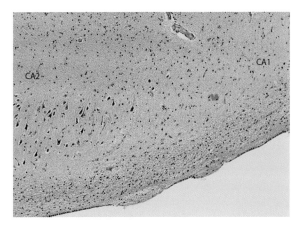

Figure 11.3 Hippocampal sclerosis H&E stain (10× magnification) with near complete loss of neurons in CA1.

the striatum with milder involvement of the globus pallidus and substantia nigra.

11.12 Final Neuropathological Diagnosis

1. Frontotemporal lobar degeneration with TDP-43 inclusions (FTLD-TDP type A)
2. Hippocampal sclerosis
3. Mild Alzheimer-type pathology

11.13 Genetic Testing

Because of the presence of ubiquitinated inclusions found in this case, the specimen was sent for genetic research screening, which showed a 90_91 ins CTGC mutation in the progranulin gene.

Re-analysis of the patient's brother's autopsy also demonstrated the presence of TDP-43 immunoreactive neuronal intranuclear inclusions in the neocortex. Therefore this case was also revised as FTLD-TDP type A, with minor AD pathology.

11.14 Discussion

Frontotemporal lobar degeneration (FTLD) is the second most common cause of dementia in individuals younger than 65 years.[1] It is a genetically complex disease, with some cases showing Mendelian inheritance pattern, while some were without a clear inheritance pattern, and others appear to be sporadic.[2] Approximately, 40% of FTLD is familial and between 10 and 15% of patients show an autosomal dominant inheritance pattern.[3,4] Of the autosomal dominant

inheritance, the most three common mutations are associated with mutations in microtubule-associated protein tau (*MAPT*), progranulin (*GRN*), and the chromosome 9 open reading frame 72 (*C9ORF72*).[5]

Progranulin is located 1.7 Mb centromeric to the *MAPT* gene on chromosome 17q21.31 and encodes a 68.5-kDa secreted growth factor involved in the regulation of multiple processes including development, wound repair, and inflammation.[5] FTLD-GRN accounts for 5–10% of all FTLD and 10–24% of familial FTLD.[6] Seventy to ninety percent of mutation carriers have a family history of dementia, and the clinical presentation can be quite heterogeneous. The mean age of onset was between 59 and 65 years, but the range varies from 35 to 89 years.[6] Disease duration varies from 3 to 22 years with a mean of 9 years.[7] Changes in behavior especially apathy and social withdrawal remains as the most common presentation; however, psychiatric symptoms such as hallucinations, delusions, and obsessive behaviors may also be seen.[5] FTLD-GRN can mimic Alzheimer's disease as seen in our case by presenting with early prominent episodic memory impairment (10–30%) combined with some evidence of apraxia, dyscalculia, and visuospatial dysfunction.[6] Extrapyramidal features can also be present in 40–60% of cases with *GRN* mutation.[7] In our case, there was a strong family history of an autosomal dominant inheritance and a faster rate of decline not typically seen in AD, raising the suspicion of a genetic cause of disease.

Neuropathologically, the most consistent feature of FTLD-GRN is the presence of ubiquitin-immunoreactive lentiform neuronal intranuclear inclusions (NII) in the neocortex and striatum.[8] Presence of neuronal cytoplasmic inclusions (NCI) and/or neuritic changes in the cerebral cortex can also be seen. It is also common to see the presence of hippocampal sclerosis in *GRN* mutations (33%). The findings observed in our case are typical in FTLD-GRN.

11.15 Take-Home Message

In cases presenting with episodic memory impairment mimicking Alzheimer's disease and having a strong family history of autosomal dominant dementia as well as a faster rate of decline and shorter disease duration, it is reasonable to consider FTLD with progranulin mutation and perform genetic screening. Interestingly, coexistence of AD pathology may have influenced the amnestic presentation of this case.

References

1. Ratnavalli E, Brayne C, Dawson K, Hodges JR. The prevalence of frontotemporal dementia. *Neurology*. 2002;58 (11):1615–1621.

2. Chen-Plotkin A, Martinez-Lage M, Sleiman P, et al. Genetic and clinical features of progranulin-associated frontotemporal lobar degeneration. *Arch Neurol*. 2011;68(4):488–497.

3. Goldman JS, Farmer JM, Wood EM, et al. Comparison of family histories in FTLD subtypes and related tauopathies. *Neurology*. 2005;65:1817–1819.

4. Rohrer JD, Guerreiro R, Vandrovcova J, et al. The heritability and genetics of frontotemporal lobar degeneration. *Neurology*. 2009;73:1451–1456.

5. Woollacott I, Rohrer J, The clinical spectrum of sporadic and familial forms of frontotemporal dementia. *J Neurochem*. 2016;138 (Suppl. 1):6–31.

6. Hsiung GYR, Feldman HH. GRN-related frontotemporal dementia. In: Adam MP, Ardinger HH, Pagon RA, eds. *Gene Reviews*. Seattle, WA: University of Washington; 1993. www.ncbi.nlm .nih.gov/books/NBK1371/.

7. Le Ber I, Camuzat A, Hannequin D, et al. Phenotype variability in progranulin mutation carriers: a clinical, neuropsychological, imaging and genetic study. *Brain*. 2008;131:732–746.

8. Mackenzie IRA, Baker M, Pickering-Brown S, et al. The neuropathology of frontotemporal lobar degeneration caused by mutations in the progranulin gene. *Brain*. 2006;129:3081–3090.

Middle-Aged Man Concerned about His Family History

Peter Roos, Jette Stokholm, Ian Law, Peter Johannsen, and Jørgen Erik Nielsen

12.1 Main Complaint

A 53-year-old man was referred to genetic counseling due to a family history of frontotemporal dementia (FTD).

12.2 Family History

On the paternal side of the family there were several cases of early-onset dementia with behavioral symptoms, and within the family this was generally referred to as "the family illness." The disease was characterized as an autosomal dominantly inherited behavioral variant FTD (bvFTD), and the cause was found to be a single base mutation in the *CHMP2B* gene on chromosome 3 giving rise to the name FTD-3.[1,2]

The father of the patient had died at the age of 70 preceded by 4 years of possible personality changes, and the patient's older brother had developed symptoms at the age of 58. Consequently, at the time of referral, the patient was considered at 50% risk of carrying the *CHMP2B* mutation.

12.3 Clinical History

At the time of referral to genetic counseling, no symptoms were apparent to either the patient or his spouse. They were however both very keen on pre-symptomatic testing. When a disease-causing mutation in the *CHMP2B* gene was confirmed, he reacted with an expectedly calm concern. He understood that the genetic predisposition did not imply an ongoing disease, and he agreed to annual evaluations at the Memory Clinic. As FTD-3 shows complete penetrance, the finding of the disease-causing mutation predicted an onset of disease no later than the age of 70.

Always a pleasant and social man, at the age of 56 he experienced difficulties handling customers at work, and he turned short tempered. He reportedly lacked initiative and structure in work performances. His general practitioner referred him to evaluation at a local psychiatrist, and a diagnosis of depression was established. When treated with antidepressants, he experienced a period of ill-considered decisions and excessive purchases of needless things, almost bordering a manic episode. One year later psychiatric evaluation showed no signs of depression and treatment was terminated. He returned to his usual tasks at work and was as always a caring husband.

In the year following this depressive episode, he would often be extremely talkative, which was considered a natural part of his extrovert personality. However, he would sometimes talk rudely to his daughter, which was unusual for him.

These minor symptoms were understated by the patient himself, but his wife expressed concern of the onset of FTD. Eighteen months after the onset of depressive symptoms, a systematic diagnostic work-up was initiated at the Memory Clinic.

12.4 General History

The patient had 15 years of education with a degree in commerce and worked in mortgage lending. He was married and had three grown-up children.

In his 20s he had been treated with steroids for pulmonary sarcoidosis. In his 30s he had suffered a minor head trauma leading to a few weeks of absence from work. He had no other former medical history. He had never smoked and had prior to referral never abused alcohol.

12.5 Examination

At the age of 57, diagnostic evaluation was initiated upon his wife's request. At this point the patient appeared short tempered but had no complaints or concerns about disease. Physical examination was unremarkable with notably no frontal release signs.

Upon psychiatric evaluation in the Memory Clinic the conversation was characterized by digressions and lack of structure. The patient presented slight psychomotor agitation, though not actual disinhibition.

At this point it was concluded that even though a depressive and subsequent manic episode had occurred in the previous year, they had ended, and there were no current psychiatric symptoms. Onset of FTD could however not be ruled out.

Neuropsychological testing found slight impairment in working memory and attention. Word mobilization was below expectancy. Rey's complex figure was constructed somewhat sloppy, and he made two errors on Trail Making test-B. Though having no problems presenting hypernyms, he did have difficulties interpreting proverbs. In the emotional hexagon he could not recognize disgust and anger. In the Iowa Gambling Task he could not comprehend the simple rules but developed idiosyncratic strategies. Overall the neuropsychological testing was inconclusive, indicating either onset of FTD or remnants from a manic episode.

[18F]fluorodeoxyglucose positron emission tomography (FDG PET)/computed tomography (CT) imaging showed reduced metabolism inferiorly in both parietal lobes and posteriorly in both temporal lobes, and slightly reduced in the mesial frontal lobe. Changes were most distinct in the right hemisphere. These findings were more suggestive of Alzheimer's disease than of FTD (Figure 12.1).

Additional work-up found normal markers of amyloid and tau in cerebrospinal fluid and no significant cortical accumulation of amyloid on 11C-PiB PET imaging. DaT scan was borderline abnormal with reduced uptake in the lentiform nucleus.

12.6 Diagnosis

The concern for onset of disease had initially been raised by his wife, and even though the previously identified *CHMP2B* mutation would suggest the obvious diagnosis of FTD-3, neuropsychological and radiological findings were uncharacteristic and failed to meet diagnostic criteria at that time. Of particular importance was the possible differential diagnosis of depression. The patient had effects from antidepressants, and indeed it was considered important to rule out this treatable and reversible disorder before settling on an untreatable diagnosis.

However, within the following year the symptoms progressed rather rapidly, the patient lacking judgment and presenting disinhibited behavior. He would offend friends and relatives to such a degree that they would avoid him, and he developed daily intake of alcohol. He soon lost the ability to perform adequately at work and lost his job. He spent excessively, buying for instance a tractor and a motortruck. He did not share his wife's concerns about expenses, and overall displayed a lack of empathy and insight.

Upon neuropsychological follow-up it was virtually impossible to have a conversation with the patient, as he would digress, fool around, or explain away any symptoms that his wife would report. Examination was described as "chaotic."

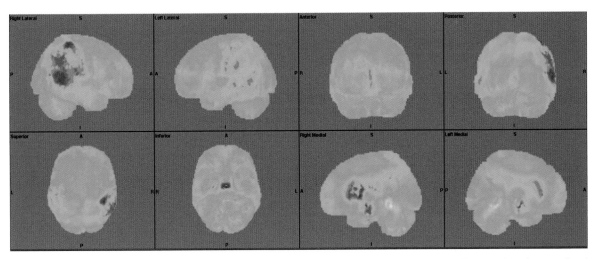

Figure 12.1 Statistical surface projections of FDG PET: At the onset of symptoms, reduced metabolism was found in the right parietal and temporal cortex, not unlike findings in Alzheimer's disease.

At this time he fulfilled the diagnostic criteria for frontotemporal dementia, and the diagnosis of FTD-3 was finally given.

12.7 Follow-Up

Five years later the patient's speech was reduced to mainly short sentences. At times he could express sadness and ascribe difficulties to "this damn disease." Though he had not been able to drive for some time, he proudly proclaimed that at his 63rd birthday he would hand in his driver's license, thus presenting some insight to his disease.

Apart from a slight bradykinesia he presented no extrapyramidal features. Occasionally fasciculation's were noticeable on the trunk and lower extremities.

Formal neuropsychological reassessment was abandoned as most tasks led to digressions of conversation. For instance, when asked to remember a name and address, he would state that he did not know anyone of that name. He could produce only four animal names before he would associate freely. The three-step Luria motor task was performed with perseveration. Visuoconstructional skills were lacking. Overall he presented with globally impaired cognitive function with executive skills most severely damaged.

When 18F-FDG PET/MRI was performed 5 years after symptom onset, atrophy of parietal and frontal lobes was apparent, and metabolism was globally reduced, now drastically involving frontal and temporal lobes (Figure 12.2).

DaT scan 5 years after onset was clearly abnormal with reduced density in the caudate nucleus, though unchanged in the lentiform nucleus. Cerebrospinal fluid (CSF) testing and PiB PET were not repeated as the patient at this time was uncooperative.

At the age of 63 the patient was institutionalized at a nursing home. He would be agreeable in familiar environments but did not tolerate changes in staff or fellow residents, and would react with aggressive and threatening behavior. It was deemed necessary to initiate antipsychotics. He soon lost his way around the institution and he isolated himself from fellow residents. Language was reduced to cliché-like phrases, though some spontaneous shorter sentences could be produced. Memory and the ability to recognize relatives were spared for a long time, while recollection of recent events deteriorated. One year later he would reluctantly use cutlery and had lost the ability to use the toilet.

Upon the latest visit, he recognized and greeted the examiner and agreed to a short walk. Gait was hypokinetic and small paced with episodes of hesitation. Language was severely reduced to short phrases, and he would repeat the words "lights-out" in a perseverating manner. Though obviously having lost all insight in his deficits, this last phrase may have been a possible expression of a former statement that he would prefer suicide to further progression of the illness.

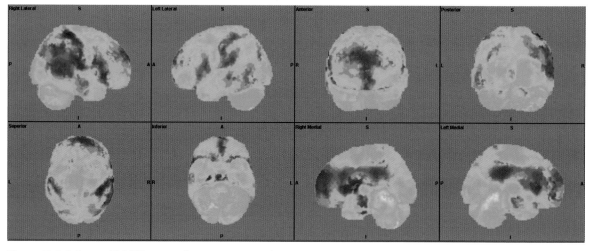

Figure 12.2 Follow-up FDG PET 5 years after symptom onset shows globally reduced metabolism.

12.8 Discussion

Frontotemporal dementia (FTD) is the second most common form of early-onset dementia after Alzheimer's disease. In the bvFTD, changes in personality are an early core feature. Patients will present disinhibited and inappropriate behavior in social relations, in language, in economic spending, and in consumption of food and alcohol. Irresponsible driving, hypersexuality, compulsive gambling, or alcohol abuse are examples of early symptoms difficult to differentiate from personality traits. Judgment and self-awareness will be altered resulting in poor decision-making. Apathy and loss of empathy is also often featured at an early stage of disease.

As illustrated by this case, in the early phases of the disease, FTD may mimic depression, mania, or other psychiatric disorders. As these are common illnesses, behavioral disturbances better accounted for by a psychiatric diagnosis are exclusionary criteria for bvFTD.[3]

However, the presence of socially inappropriate behavior or the loss of empathy and insight should alert the clinician to the possible diagnosis of FTD. Due to the anosognosia of the patient, information from relatives is almost mandatory in revealing tactlessness and the breaking of social rules. As subtle symptoms may be personality traits, the history should include ongoing changes and progression compared to earlier behavior.

At this point neuropsychological profiling is helpful in diagnostics. Test results may be normal in the early phases of primarily behavioral changes, but the finding of executive deficits will be helpful. Testing may also reveal perseveration or lack of judgment and of abstraction. Memory can be spared.

As the disease progresses, symptoms become manifest evolving into incontrollable impulsiveness or complete inertia. Executive functions will decline with loss of functional activities and a more pronounced dementia.

Motor function will deteriorate, and patients can exhibit extra pyramidal features or motor neuron involvement.

There is neither curative nor palliative treatment for FTD.

Most cases of FTD are sporadic, but in as many as 40% there is a family history of similar disease, often in an autosomal dominant inheritance pattern. A number of disease-causing mutations have been identified in genes such as *MAPT, GRN, C9orf72, FUS, VCP, TARDP-43*, and – as in this case – *CHMP2B*.[4] Consequently, presence of a known pathogenic mutation is an important factor in the diagnostic criteria for FTD.[3]

While the presymptomatic finding of a disease-causing mutation would guide the physician in the diagnostic process, the patient presented here should demonstrate the challenges when facing a disease of personality changes.

In this case symptom onset was preceded by 1 year of depression. When treated, the patient returned to his previous skills and personality for a short period of time. Initial symptoms were minor executive difficulties and short temper followed by an almost manic episode of careless spending. Bipolar disorder would be an obvious diagnosis, and also an important one to consider, as bipolar disorder – unlike FTD – is treatable and potentially reversible. Thorough evaluation was performed before excluding psychiatric disease. And even though FTD was expected to appear in this genetically verified carrier of the *CHMP2B* mutation, a specific time of onset was difficult to establish.

The following rather rapid progression of symptoms precipitated as obvious bvFTD. In less than 2 years the patient fulfilled diagnostic criteria in a discouraging fashion.

Follow-up neuropsychology confirmed an almost global affection of cognition, while functional imaging substantiated the progression of the neurodegenerative process.

12.9 Take-Home Messages

Neurodegenerative diseases are characterized by progression of symptoms. While an exact time of onset is difficult to establish, the progression will most often reveal the diagnosis.

Early symptoms of frontotemporal dementia may be subtle changes in behavior misinterpreted as depression or other psychiatric disease.

Treatable or reversible diagnoses should be taken into serious consideration when facing the otherwise obvious diagnostics of an untreatable or irreversible condition.

Furthermore, in the case of familial non-treatable disorders the patient's and the family's wishes in relation to presymptomatic testing and subsequent clinical diagnosis should be taken into careful consideration.

References

1. Gydesen S, Brown JM, Brun A, et al. Chromosome 3 linked frontotemporal dementia (FTD-3). *Neurology.* 2002;59:1585–1594.

2. Skibinski G, Parkinson NJ, Brown JM, et al. Mutations in the endosomal ESCRTIII-complex subunit CHMP2B in frontotemporal dementia. *Nat Genet.* 2005;37: 806–808.

3. Rascovsky K, Hodges JR, Knopman D, et al. Sensitivity of revised diagnostic criteria for the behavioural variant of frontotemporal dementia. *Brain.* 2011;134:2456–2477.

4. Paulson HL, Igo I. Genetics of dementia. *Semin Neurol.* 2011;31:449–460.

Man Having Trouble Reading

Bruno F. A. L. Franchi and Ashan Khurram

13.1 Clinical History – Main Complaint

JX is a 60-year-old man who presented to his general practitioner in mid-June of 2015 complaining that he was finding his spreadsheets at work harder to manage. He had taken a month of leave to seek medical attention. He had no difficulties describing the content of the spreadsheets to his colleagues, but found he had to zoom in on the specific pieces of data to be able to see them. He noted if he intently stared at the screen things would move around or change. He initially saw an opthalmologist, and there were no issues with his fields or acuity. He stated straight lines appeared crooked or had "knuckles" on them.

His wife noticed the occasional difficulty grasping new mental concepts or interpretating what an object in front of him was. Number recognition could be difficult. She noted the issues first started 4 years ago, had been slowly progressive, but was not affecting his work until recently.

He described accompanying lethargy and some weight loss despite not changing his lifestyle.

13.2 General History

JX has a year 10 education and works in a very demanding position involving the electronic statewide logistic coordination of fire service assets in a highly fire-prone state. His medical history is only significant for obstructive sleep apnea (which responded to a jaw splint). He lives with his wife and has two healthy children.

He has no regular medications. He drinks 10–20 g of alcohol a day.

He has never smoked and has no history of hypertension, diabetes, or hypercholesterolemia.

13.3 Family History

His mother is currently alive with a diagnosis of probable Alzheimer's disease. No other significant family history.

13.4 Examination

BP 130/80, pulse 70 regular, chest was clear, and there was no significant adenopathy or organomegaly.

Cranial nerve examination was normal, as was peripheral nerve testing. There was no evidence of cerebellar dysfunction, nor signs of parkinsonism. There were no clinical frontal release signs. His gait was unremarkable.

Foldstein's Mini-Mental State Examination (MMSE): 27/30 (lost one point in orientation, one with recall and significant difficulty with construction, failing to copy one pentagram). Clock face drawing was significantly impaired. Frontal Assessment Battery score: 17/18 (one point lost in mental flexibility). The score was 3/15 on the Geriatric Depression Scale (indicating low probability of depression).

13.5 Special Studies

MRI head – moderate bilateral parietal lobe atrophy. No temporal or hippocampal atrophy. No significant small vessel disease.

Blood results – vasculitis screen, TSH, B12, folate, HIV, syphilis serology all negative.

EEG – no abnormalities detected.

Neuropsychological testing – extremely severe visuoperceptual and visuoconstructional impairment. He was unable to put down more than a few isolated features from a complex figure (see Figure 13.1). Color identification was accurate. There may have been some mild left-sided visual neglect. There was no optic ataxia. There were several visual misperceptions (a dog's head was seen as a guitar, still struggling even when his mistake was pointed out). Reading was accurate with slight hesitancy. Writing to dictation was accurate but messy. There was some subtle bilateral finger agnosia. He described mild difficulty with dressing. There were no issues with working memory or mental arithmetic. There was no evidence of a receptive dysphasia. His executive mental flexibility was in the superior range when corrected for his poor visual tracking. Semantic and verbal fluencies were in the high average range.

SPECT scan – moderate hypoperfusion of the posterior parietal lobes, more marked on the right. Patchy hypoperfusion of the temporal lobes posterolaterally and anteromedially. Preservation of

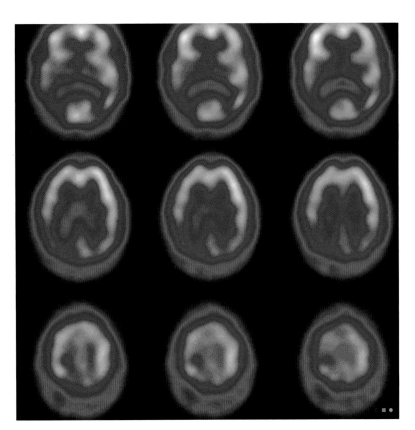

Figure 13.1 SPECT scan image demonstrating particularly right posterior parietal issues taken at JX's initial presentation.

frontal, occipital, and subcortical regions (see Figure 13.2).

A lumbar puncture was not felt to be necessary.

13.6 Diagnosis

Atypical Alzheimer's disease – posterior cortical atrophy (PCA) (Benson's syndrome).

13.7 Follow-Up

Initial management involved referral to a specialist occupational therapist for return to work strategies. Despite this he did not successfully return to work.

Formal review 18 months after initial presentation revealed rapid progression of cognitive dysfunction over multiple domains. He had lost insight into the severity of his illness.

Old repetitive tasks were completed without difficulty, such as feeding the dog. If the task was dependent on more than three steps, however, he will invariably forget one. He seemed to remember things that directly affect him, such as appointments, but promptly forgot things that did not directly involve him. He remembers faces and people (no prosopagnosia). His wife felt he can still file memories away, often retrieving them weeks later. She felt his memory issues stemmed from limited storage, with information going in at the cost of other memories (unusual in typical Alzheimer's disease).

He was easily distractible with concentration being an issue. He was usually oriented but has been lost when being driven around. His decision-making has been impaired as he struggled to appreciate how the decision will affect him.

He complained of his hands becoming cold along with increasing constipation. There were no symptoms of postural instability. His sleep had become less settled, and included two episodes of dream-related urinary incontinence. There were a few occasions where he could not find the toilet at night. His appetite

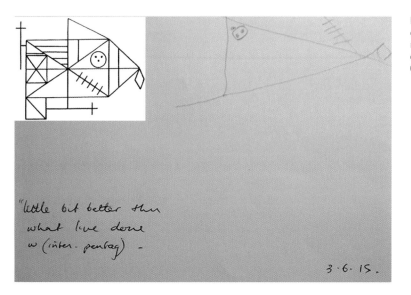

Figure 13.2 Rey diagram and that constructed by JX at initial presentation in mid-2015. https://openi.nlm.nih.gov/detailedresult.php?img=PMC3001689_PSM-07-07-g-001&req=4.

"little but better than what I've done w (inter. pentag) –

3·6·15.

increased but his weight remained stable. His taste for food had changed, having acquired a "sweet tooth" and his body shape has changed as a result (muscle loss with fat gain). His speed of eating had decreased. He did not have swallowing issues. He struggled to cut up his food related to his visuospatial issues.

His wife suggested he will put things upside down more than 90% of the time. He had difficulty judging distances, often missing the table when putting down his coffee cup. Clothes are put on inside out, and he would try to put his head into the arm holes. It could take up to 1 hour to complete dressing. There were no difficulties with left/right orientation, although it could take a bit of thought and time. He had great difficulty making the bed, directly related to spatial orientation.

He had developed myoclonic jerks.

The decision was made to commence him on an acetylcholine esterase inhibitor.

He was strongly encouraged to consider donation of his brain to the South Australian Brain Bank.

13.8 Discussion

PCA (also known as Benson's syndrome) is a clinical presentation of neurodegenerative disorders. Although the majority of cases are related to underlying Alzheimer's disease, a small but significant number are related to Dementia with Lewy Bodies (DLB), Corticobasal Degeneration (CBD), or underlying Prion disease. Ultimately, it is the accompanying clues in the clinical presentation that can help differentiate the underlying pathology. Although there are not enough cases or trials to dictate treatment measures, a strong clinical suspicion for Alzheimer's disease should be upheld and consideration of the merits of acetylcholine esterase treatment undertaken.

A recent review article of PCA published in *Lancet Neurology* provides a cogent summary of the current understanding of the presenting features of this syndrome. It tends not to be sex specific, it occurs generally in a younger cohort (55–60), and is (mostly) part of a spectrum of unusual presentations of Alzheimer's disease. One set of diagnostic criterion include (i) insidious onset and gradual progression, (ii) presentation of visual deficits in the absence of ocular disease, (iii) relatively preserved episodic memory, verbal fluency and personal insight, (iv) presence of symptoms including visual agnosia, simultanagnosia, optic ataxia, ocular apraxia, dyspraxia and environmental disorientation, and (v) absence of stroke or tumor.[1] Our clinical case is presented in a fashion that fulfills these criterion.

Although some cases of PCA can present with other features of parietal lobe dysfunction (e.g.,

Gerstmann's syndrome – left/right disorientation, acalculia, agraphia, finger agnosia), JX initially clinically was able to perform these functions when it was not a visually dependent task. He did not initially have features that fulfilled Balint's syndrome (oculomotor apraxia, simultanagnosia, or optic ataxia) although as his disease progressed these components were very likely to be contributing to his poor daily function. As the disease progresses toward a global dementia state, often anterograde memory, executive functions, and linguistic skills become affected.[1]

The initial visual disturbances JX described fit well with the understanding of patients with PCA complaints. Often, basic visual disturbances are described (form, motion, color, point localization). His perception of the movement of static stimuli, and 180° upside-down reversal of vision have been described. Other features he did not exhibit include abnormally prolonged color after images and the reverse size phenomenon. One cohort of PCA patients (investigated with fMRI) had issues with stereopsis, saccadic eye movements, and higher functional impairments (simultanagnosia, image orientation, figure-from-ground segregation, closure, and spatial orientation).[2] Ventral visual regions (face and object perception) were preserved whereas more dorsal areas were impaired.

Simultanagnosia is the inability to see multiple visual objects at the same time. When examining the specific visual process difficulties in patients affected by PCA there was a slowing of visual processing speed with preserved visual short-term memory.[3]

Myoclonus has been described in one case series in 24% of people affected by PCA. JX's rapid eye movement sleep disturbance may hint at a Lewy body process; however, the autonomic issues may be related to Corticobasal degeneration. There were no prominent frontal signs clinically (26% of PCA's can have a positive grasp reflex) yet some of the history findings (appetite changes, loss of insight, difficulty weighing up decisions) may suggest some impairment.[4] Ultimately his follow-up supported a global neurodegenerative process.

Neuroimaging is useful in helping to determine the underlying pathological cause of the PCA syndrome. When compared to patients with early Alzheimer's disease those with PCA have a higher mean hippocampal volume,[5] while the bilateral hypometabolic pattern on PET scanning involved posterior, temporal, and occipital cortex (especially the right parieto-occipital cortex).[6] Calculation and visuospatial abilities were correlated with this cortical volume.[5] On PET scanning, patterns of glucose utilization were similar between DLB and PCA with some subtle differences in the patterns.[7]

The greater than 4-year history is against a prion process.

It is unlikely that his family history is important – further questioning suggested his mother's illness was much later in life, more typical for Alzheimer's disease in features and slowly progressive over more than 10 years. Case series publications do not support a strong family history of Alzheimer's disease in those with PCA[1] although several recent publications have suggested important genetic loci.[8,9]

13.9 Take-Home Messages

1. A predominantly visual symptom presentation in younger patients can be Alzheimer's related
2. Neuroimaging patterns in unusual presentations of neurodegenerative disorders can help to differentiate the underlying pathological cause

References

1. Crutch SJ, Lehmann M, Schott JM, et al. Posterior cortical atrophy. *Lancet Neurol.* 2012;11:170–178.

2. Shames H, Raz N, Levin N. Functional neural substrates of posterior cortical atrophy patients. *J Neurol.* 2015;262:1751–1761.

3. Neitzel J, Ortner M, Haupt M, et al., Neuro-cognitive mechanisms of simultanagnosia in patients with posterior cortical atrophy. *Brain.* 2016;139:3267–3280.

4. Snowden JS, Stopford CL, Julien CL, et al. Cognitive phenotypes in Alzheimer's disease and genetic risk. *Cortex.* 2007;43:835–845.

5. Peng G, Wang J, Feng Z, et al., Clinical and neuroimaging differences between posterior cortical atrophy and typical amnestic Alzheimer's disease patients at an early disease stage. *Sci Rep.* 2016;6:29372.

6. Cerami C, Crespi C, Della Rosa PA, et al. Brain changes within the visuo-spatial attentional network in posterior cortical

atrophy. *J Alzheimers Dis.* 2015;43:385–395.

7. Whitwell J, Graff-Radford J, Singh T, et al. ^{18}F-FDG PET in posterior cortical atrophy and dementia with Lewy bodies. *J Nucl Med.* 2016;58(4):632–638.

8. Schott JM, Crutch SJ, Carrasquillo MM, et al. Genetic risk factors for the posterior cortical atrophy variant of Alzheimer's disease. *Alzheimers Dement.* 2016;12: 862–871.

9. Carrasquillo MM, Barber I, Lincoln SJ, et al. Evaluating pathogenic dementia variants in posterior cortical atrophy. *Neurobiol Aging.* 2016;37: 38–44.

Speechless at First Sight

Marie-Pierre Thibodeau and Fadi Massoud

14.1 Case History

A 66-year-old right-handed man presented to the memory clinic with a complaint of decreased concentration.

He was of Portuguese descent, highly educated and was retired from employment in airport security. He spoke three languages fluently. He lived with his second wife and was active and independent in his activities of daily living. His wife had always been responsible for house chores, but the patient managed his finances and drove without major difficulties. He had however been released from his job for unclear reasons 5 years earlier.

Past medical history only included benign prostate hypertrophy and recent surgery for inguinal hernia. He had no personal or family history of neurological or mental conditions. There was no history of alcohol or drug abuse.

The patient's spontaneous complaint was of decreased concentration while reading for the past 3 years. Upon further questioning it was found that he had difficulty interpreting what was on the paper; he needed to turn his head in a specific position to read and got easily tired. His attention and memory were preserved when he managed to read adequately. He also drove more slowly for fear of not reacting fast enough to upcoming visual obstacles. He was reported driving at 30 km/h on small roads because of this fear of hitting a child or an animal. His wife described symptoms of simultagnosia, the patient having difficulties finding objects in cluttered spaces such as the refrigerator or cupboard. He also reported problems putting a key in a keyhole or pouring wine in a glass. He had no disorientation in space or time, and his memory was globally preserved. At the time of the first evaluation the patient reported also some very mild word finding difficulty that gradually increased on follow-up. He was also described as being more anxious without any other behavioral change. He described his vision as being normal. He had no hallucinations or delusions, and no other neurological symptoms were reported.

14.2 Physical Examination

Throughout history and physical examination the patient was eager to perform, anxious and overly appreciative of the care he was given. On physical examination significant difficulties copying finger movements on visual cues, but not on verbal cues were noted. He easily pretended to comb his hair or brush his teeth, but was unable to imitate the examiner taping his fingers or making hand signs. He had agraphesthesia without astereognosia bilaterally. Cranial nerves, strength, reflexes, and cerebellar function were normal. He had no parkinsonism or gait problems.

14.3 Cognitive Examination

On cognitive examination, visuoperceptual difficulties were mainly noted. He was unable to copy the pentagons on the Mini-Mental State Examination (MMSE) and his clock drawing was inadequate. While describing the cookie jar figure he was unable to see the global picture or to identify specific objects because of visual interference. The Navon letter test was abnormal. He had right-left agnosia, dyslexia, and dysgraphia. At first, mild anomia was noted and seemed mainly related to his visuoperceptual problems. He had no speech apraxia, dysarthria, agrammatism, or semantic loss. Memory was spared.Neuropsychological examination revealed simultagnosia, left hemi-inattention, left-right distinction vulnerability, construction and ideomotor apraxia, alexia, agraphia, lexical access problems, and decreased executive functions with preserved verbal memory and behavior.

The patient was sent for an ophthalmological examination that revealed right homonymous hemianopsia.

A brain scan was performed and showed mild atrophy and leurcoaraiosis without any mass. A PET scan was also performed and revealed severe parietal hypoperfusion bilaterally more on the left than the right and mild temporal hypo metabolism bilaterally L>R (Figure 14.1).

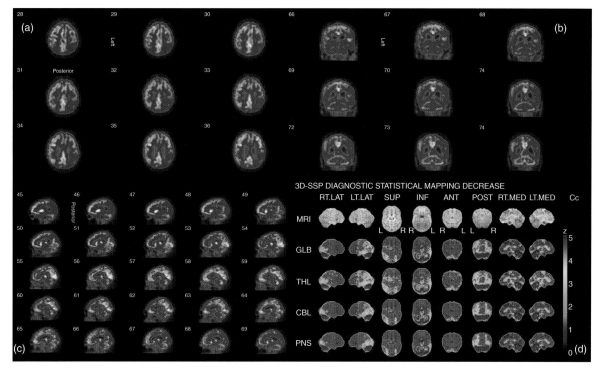

Figure 14.1 [^{18}F]FDG PET study. Transaxial (a), coronal (b), and sagittal slices (radiological orientation, right side of subject on the left side of the figure) showing severely diminished metabolism in parietal and occipital regions (left worse than right), with mild extension into the posterior region of the left temporal lobe. Prefrontal associative cortices remain normal. The posterior portions of the cingulate gyri also show normal distribution (c). 3D-SSP representation confirms that pattern (d).

14.4 Diagnosis

A diagnosis of posterior cortical Atrophy (PCA) was given with associated logopenia. Treatment with donepezil was initiated.

14.5 Follow-Up

As the disease progressed, the patient developed more severe word-finding difficulty. Naming common objects became difficult with use of multiple nonspecific words in conversations as well as periphrases. Semantic knowledge was preserved. Sense of direction became more impaired and the patient started progressively losing his short-term memory. He still remained active and functioned well in his daily activities.

14.6 Discussion

PCA is a neurodegenerative disease dominated by impairment in visuospatial and visuoperceptual functions. Characteristic features of PCA include Balint's syndrome (simultanagnosia; optic ataxia [impaired visually guided grasping]; ocular apraxia [impaired voluntary saccades to visual targets]; environmental agnosia); and Gerstmann's syndrome (agraphia, acalculia, right-left confusion, and finger agnosia). Components of both syndromes are found only partially in most patients. Additionally, there may be visual agnosia, alexia with or without agraphia, anomia, environmental disorientation, apraxia, hemi-inattention, prosopagnosia, and aphasia. All of these elements are rarely found as a whole at first but can appear as disease spreads throughout the brain.[1]

These very variable clinical features contribute to the confusion surrounding the diagnosis of PCA and to its often delayed diagnosis. The urgency to develop well recognized clinical diagnostic criteria has been emphasized by an expert consortium following the International Conference on Alzheimer's and related dementias in 2012.[2] Insidious onset and gradual

Table 14.1 Proposed key features of PCA

Cardinal features
- Insidious onset and gradual progression
- Prominent visuoperceptual/visuospatial impairment with relatively preserved ophthalmic examination
- Complex visual dysfunction
- Absent stroke or tumor
- Preserved memory and insight

Supportive features
- Alexia
- Presenile onset
- Ideomotor/dressing apraxia
- Prosopagnosia
- Prolonged color after-images

Based on Crutch et al.[2]

progression, prominent visuoperceptual/visuospatial impairment with relatively preserved ophthalmic examination, complex visual dysfunction, absent stroke or tumor, and preserved memory and insight are cardinal features according to this international working group. Alexia, presenile onset, ideomotor/dressing apraxia, prosopagnosia, prolonged color after-images (persistence of an image after exposure) are proposed supportive features (Table 14.1). However, future criteria that will ensure a more precise diagnosis should be elaborated following collaborative work.

Simultagnosia (the inability to perceive a global picture despite seeing all the components) is the most commonly found complex visual dysfunction and explains most patients' difficulties with reading and daily functioning. It can be easily identified at bedside with the cookie-jar figure and Navon letter (e.g., a big H made from small Vs). Many other phenomena may explain reading difficulties such as visual disorientation (getting lost on the page), reverse size phenomena (accurately perceiving small but not large print), and visual crowding.

The underlying pathology in more than 80% of patients is Alzheimer's disease (AD) explaining why PCA is often called an atypical form of AD or posterior AD.[3] As opposed to classic AD, patients with PCA are younger at onset and have preserved memory and insight. As a consequence of this, patients often develop significant anxiety more so than typical AD. This anxiety can be so important that it can mislead even experienced clinicians to

diagnosing a psychological problem rather than PCA. Other pathologies to consider are Lewy bodies and corticobasal degeneration (CBD). In this case, AD was most probable because of the age of onset, prominent visuoperceptual impairment without parkinsonism or hallucinations suggestive of Lewy body dementia. Corticobasal degeneration was not supported by imaging and the nature of the aphasia was not of the nonfluent type usually associated with CBD.

A few studies have reported a language profile in PCA that is similar the logopenic variant of primary progressive aphasia (LPA).[4] Language disorders were reported in the first description of PCA by Benson, but later neglected in subsequent studies. Patients with PCA typically have anomia and reduced phonemic fluency as dominant language features. Compared to LPA, the aphasic syndrome in PCA is milder and exhibits more impairment in single-word retrieval and working memory while speech production is more preserved. The left temporo-parietal junction seems to play an important role in the logopenic syndrome. As the disease progresses it is logical to expect spread to contiguous brain areas as seen in this patient.

Homonymous hemianopsia has also been reported in PCA in up to 50–100% of cases. It is however often underdiagnosed because patients are not referred to ophthalmologists or the latter do not refer patients to memory clinics. Associated symptoms are related to higher visual functions such as simultagnosia and hemi-inattention.[5]

All patients with suspected PCA should undergo ophthalmological examination and brain imaging with scan or MRI to rule out an underlying anatomic lesion. When available PET imaging will show bilateral occipito-parietal hypo-metabolism. In the case presented here, the underlying pathological process is likely Alzheimer's disease despite normal uptake in the posterior portions of the cingulate gyri on PET, as variant presentations of Alzheimer's can present with delayed hypometabolism in those areas. PIB-PET is usually amyloid positive. Neuropsychological evaluation may help underscore the prominent visuoperceptual impairment with preserved verbal memory and insight.

Very few therapeutic studies have be conducted with patients with PCA. There is, in fact, no evidence-based data showing efficacy of cholinesterase inhibitors for PCA. However, because of the presumed cholinergic deficit, cholinesterase inhibitors can be expected to have beneficial effects in patients with Alzheimer's or Lewy body pathologies. It is of common practice to offer this treatment to patients. Referral to resources for the visually impaired should also be considered.

The longitudinal course of the disease has rarely been reported. Progressive decline is expected in other cortical functions as the disease spreads throughout the brain, with patients gradually displaying more typical symptoms of AD.

References

1. Borruat FX. Posterior cortical atrophy: review of recent literature. *Curr Neurol Neurosci Rep*. 2013;13:406–408.

2. Crutch SJ, Schott JM, Rabinovici GD, et al. Shining a light on posterior cortical atrophy. *Alzheimers Dement.* 2013;9:463–465.

3. Crutch S, Lehmann M, Schott JM, et al. Posterior cortical atrophy. *Lancet Neurol.* 2012;11:170–178.

4. Crutch S, Lehmann M, Warren JD, Rohrer JD. The language profile of posterior cortical atrophy. *J Neural Neurosurg Psychiatry.* 2013;84:460–466.

5. Beh SC, Muthusamy B, Calabresi P, et al. Hiding in plain sight: a closer look at posterior cortical atrophy. *Pract Neurol.* 2015;15:5–13.

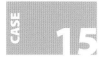

From Stuttering to Mutism

Thais Helena Machado, Elisa de Paula França Resende,
Henrique Cerqueira Guimarães, and Maria Teresa Carthery-Goulart

15.1 Clinical History – Main Complaint

EEP is a Brazilian, 68-year-old, right-handed man, with 15 years of schooling (graduated in business school). He is married and has a daughter and a son.

Now retired, he had worked for many years in his own real estate business. His main work-related activities involved sales and purchase of land, which were accomplished with the help of an office assistant.

At the age of 63 his wife noticed that at times when trying to express himself, EEP presented with difficulties characterized by pauses and stuttering episodes. Although this fact had been pointed by her to him, initially EEP did not care enough for these symptoms and did not find it necessary to seek medical advice. Over the following 3 years symptoms have gradually become worse and in some occasions his speech was blocked and word-finding difficulties also emerged. At that time, he decided to seek medical advice. His main complaint was about speech production, characterized by fluency problems (pauses and prosodic changes, including hesitations and stuttering). His wife also had noticed word-finding difficulties, including reading and writing activities.

Despite those speech and language problems EEP continued working (with the help of his assistant), driving a vehicle properly, and did not present with memory or any other cognitive complaints. Functional performance in activities of daily living was preserved except for those involving language. Social activities had been gradually reduced as expression problems became worse.

15.2 General History

The patient was healthy, with no reported comorbidities. He had no history of developmental learning or language problems, previous psychiatric or neurological problems. In his free time, he had a busy social agenda, engaging in several meetings with friends and also in sport activities. He had been a nonprofessional athlete for over 30 years, did not smoke, and had healthy diet habits. His mood was good at that first evaluation, and no behavioral changes could be emphasized. Depressive symptoms emerged just when the patient become aware of his difficulties, in a moderate stage of impairment.

15.3 Family History

Only his father and a distant aunt had memory difficulties after 80s.

15.4 Examination

15.4.1 Neurological Exam

His neurological exam was normal, without motor or sensory deficit or equilibrium impairment. Only cognitive impairment was detected.

15.4.2 Neuropsychological Evaluation

EEP scored 27/30 in the Mini-Mental State Examination (MMSE), 12/18 in the Frontal Assessment Battery, 11/30 in forward and backward digit span (WAIS III battery) and 49″ and 144″ in the Trails test parts A and B, respectively.

Combined, those neuropsychological tests pointed to a mild impairment of executive functions, including phonological short-term memory and working memory difficulties. Other cognitive functions were preserved. He was oriented in time and space (MMSE), nonverbal episodic memory tests were within the normal range and autobiographical memory also seemed preserved. According to his wife, he was independent and functional for basic and instrumental activities of daily living, except for more complex administrative and financial tasks, in which he showed a progressively increased need for assistance with more marked difficulties appearing in the previous year (2 years after the onset of speech symptoms).

15.4.3 Speech and Language Assessment

Speech and language was assessed in a functional communicative evaluation (semi-structured interview) and also with formal tests. In the functional situation, auditory comprehension was quite well preserved as well as pragmatic resources (suitable communicative exchange shifts, maintenance of eye contact and nonverbal communication). On the other hand, oral production was marked by anomia, word-finding difficulties, and large quantity of pauses between words and sentences. Moreover, there was important output reduction, characterized by short and simplified sentences with omission of verbs and function words (i.e., prepositions, conjunctions, etc.), as well as substitutions of verb inflections. Speech was effortful, slow, and hesitant. Occasional phonemic paraphasias (omission and substitutions of phonemes) were also observed. Mild prosodic changes (intonation, stress, and rhythm) were also present. The results of the main language tests employed in the formal speech and language assessment are as follows (Table 15.1):

- *Oral and Buccofacial Praxis*: The patient had no difficulty with nonverbal agility, however he manifested mild apraxia of speech in tests of verbal agility and diadochokinesia test.
- *Oral Naming*: EEP produced spontaneously 35/60 correct responses in the Boston Naming test. His responses suggested problems in lexical access with preservation of semantics. He was able to provide definitions of items he was unable to name and in most of them, when given phonemic cues (i.e., the first phoneme or syllable) he was able to produce the correct name.
- *Verbal fluency* was markedly impaired both for semantic category (animals) and for letters (FAS), although letter fluency impairment was more severe (only two items in 3 min).
- *Repetition*: The ability for short and frequent sentences was preserved. Word repetition was preserved except for longer multi-syllabic words. Phonological errors as well as word omission or semantic substitutions were observed in the repetition of low frequency and long sentences.
- *Oral picture description*: Speech and language production difficulties were evident in the oral discourse production task of Boston aphasia assessment (cookie theft picture). In this task, EEP presented *telegraphic speech*, that is, he was unable to produce long and complete sentences and expressed mainly through content words. Verb production was markedly reduced (only three verbs) and errors in verb tenses (past

Table 15.1 Performance on language tasks

Sentence comprehension	TROG	Total score 53/80
		Passed Blocks 6/20
	Token test	1ª part: 100%
		2ª part: 100%
		3ª part: 70%
		4ª part: 10%
		5ª part: 23.80%
Naming	Boston Naming Test	35/60
Verbal fluency	Animals	5
	FAS	2
Repetition	Boston Test	9/10
	Words	6/8
	Sentences with high-frequency words	4/8
	Sentences with low-frequency words	
Reading	Boston Test	30/30
	Words	7/10
	Phrases	1/25
	Reading protocol HFSP	0/7
		¾
	Regular words	
	Irregular words	
	Pseudo words	
Writing	Boston Test	3/5
	Narrative writing	2/25
	Dictation protocol HFSP	4/7
		¼
	Regular words	
	Irregular words	
	Pseudo words	

participle used instead of gerund) were also observed.

Transcription of cookie theft picture and translation:

mulher... homem... pote... mulher... prato pia vazando... caído... caído... nu nu banco... caído banco

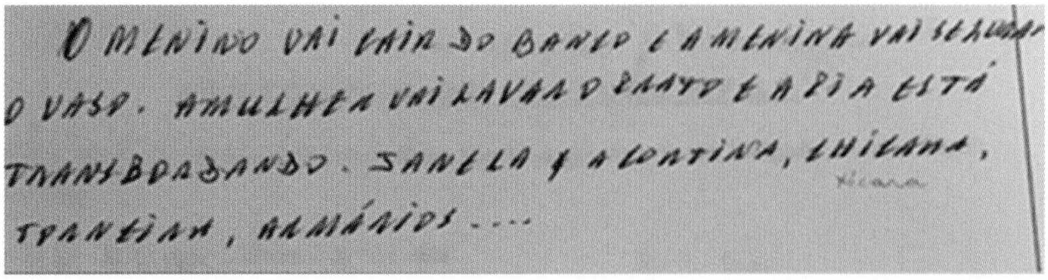

Figure 15.1 Writing description of the theft of cookies.

é:: prato... xícara... num sei o que não...
janela... cortina... pia sobrando água... planta

« woman... man... pot... woman... dish
sink leaking... fallen... fallen in the in the stock...
fallen stock
is:: dish... cup... I don't know what...
window... curtain... sink... water... plant »

Legend: ... means silent pause; :: means prolongation

- *Auditory comprehension*: This ability was preserved for words but not for sentences, as evaluated by the Token test and the Test for Reception of Grammar (TROG-2). Token test evaluates the comprehension of commands and is useful to distinguish problems with increased sentence length (Part 3) from deficits in sentences with more complex syntactic structure (Part 5). EEP results pointed out to problems related both to phonological working memory (errors with increased sentence length) as well as syntactic structure. TROG test is used to assess a range of lexical, morphosyntactic, and syntactic structures. The patient's performance in this test pointed to attentional problems (sporadic errors with some structures) as well as genuine morphosyntactic comprehension deficits in reversible constructions, zero anaphora sentences, use of pronouns (gender, number, and binding), singular/plural inflections, relative clauses, and center embedded sentences.

- *Reading*: In the patient, this ability was preserved for words (regular and irregular) and nonwords. When reading sentences he omitted and transposed phonemes, omitted articles, prepositions, and conjunctions. In spite of that, formal tests pointed to satisfactory written comprehension of sentences and short texts.

- *Writing*: An assessment pointed to occasional errors in a dictation task. These errors occurred only in words with irregular or exceptional spelling, but the ability to write nonwords was preserved, that is, the patient tends to use rules for translating phonemes in graphemes (mild surface dysgraphia).

Narrative written production was better than the oral production. In written production EEP was able to produce grammatically accurate short sentences. The cookie theft description was reduced (as in the oral output condition), but EEP was able to produce some grammatically simple sentences and lexical access to verbs was also better, as is shown in the Figure 15.1.

Translation: "the boy is going to fall from the stool and the girl is going hold the vase. The woman is going to wash the dish and the sink is overflowing. Window, curtain, cup, tap, cupboards ..."

15.4.4 Neuroimaging Findings and Biomarker Analysis

The patient also underwent lumbar puncture in order to investigate cerebrospinal fluid (CSF) biomarkers related to Alzheimer's disease (AD) (ELISA Innotest® kit). The analysis disclosed the following results: $A\beta42$ = 536.4 pg/ml, tau = 282.9 pg/ml, p-tau = 52.5 pg/ml.

15.5 Initial Diagnosis

Based on the overall clinical, neuropsychological, language, and neuroimaging data, a diagnosis of Primary Progressive Aphasia (PPA), nonfluent/agrammatic variant (PPA-A) was made.

15.6 Follow-Up

This patient was submitted to a brief behavioral intervention program, with a speech and language therapist, focusing on sentence production described elsewhere.[1] After this program, he attended rehabilitation twice a week.

Six months after the language assessment, EEP started to manifest attention deficit and impulsiveness. In the following 6 months other symptoms appeared: sleep problems and decline in functional activities (i.e., remote control or cell phone use). During this period, his verbal output worsened, with

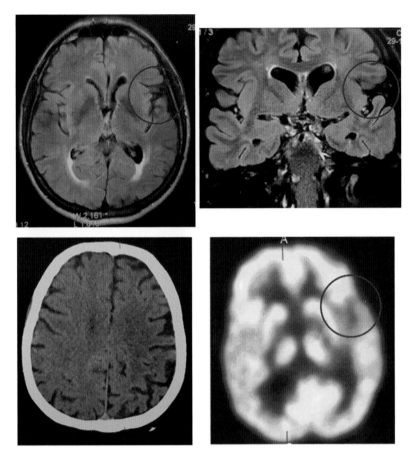

Figure 15.2 Superior row from left to right: axial and coronal Fluid Attenuated Inversion Recovery magnetic resonance imaging showing left inferior frontoinsular atrophy with anterior Sylvian fissure enlargement (red circle) and unspecific periventricular hyperintensities. Inferior row (left): high convexity axial computed tomography slice displaying asymmetric atrophy in left brain hemisphere; (right): [F18] FDG-positron emission tomography showing reduced metabolism in the posterior portion of the inferior frontal gyrus and insula (blue circle).

frequent pauses and hesitations and naming deficits also worsened.

A year and a half after the first examination, his speech output was markedly reduced (he was unable to use verbs and no sentences were produced) and oral comprehension became more impaired. Global cognitive deficits became evident. He gradually reduced the amount of work and retired soon afterward.

Two years after the diagnosis, EEP was severely aphasic, with his speech output being limited to single words and nonverbal communication. As functional losses became more evident, occupational therapy and gradually substituted speech and language intervention were included in his rehabilitation program.

Almost 6 years after his first symptoms, the patient presents severe aphasia characterized by mutism and marked comprehension deficits. Despite that, he is still partially independent for basic activities of daily living.

15.7 Discussion

EEP's symptoms denote a typical case of PPA, a clinical syndrome characterized by a predominant and progressive language deficit due to gradual neurodegeneration of the left hemisphere in critical points of the language network. This diagnosis is made when three conditions are fulfilled: most prominent clinical feature is difficulty with language; language difficulties are the main cause of impairment in every-day activities; and aphasia is the most prominent deficit at symptom onset and for the initial phases of the disease. In addition, the pattern of deficits must not be better accounted for by other neurodegenerative nervous system or psychiatric disorder.[2] In 2011, an international group of PPA investigators agreed on terminology and on clinical, imaging-supported, and definite pathology criteria for the diagnosis of three distinct PPA variants: nonfluent/agrammatic (PPA-A), semantic (PPA-S), and logopenic (PPA-L).[3]

PPA is usually an early-onset dementia, with symptoms starting before the age of 65. Early identification of PPA may be challenging in nonspecialized clinics as very mild speech and language changes may go unnoticed. In fact, EEP sought medical advice only 3 years after symptoms onset, when speech and language deficits posed marked difficulties in work and social activities. In other cases, PPA patients may receive an erroneous clinical diagnosis of Alzheimer's disease (AD). However, PPA's cognitive and imaging profile is different from other dementia syndromes. In terms of neuropsychological assessment PPA doesn't begin with prominent amnestic, behavioral, or visuospatial symptoms. Language deficits may remain as single cognitive manifestations for variable periods over the course of the disease and even when other neuropsychological deficits appear, language is the most severely affected function (for a review of the clinical symptoms of PPA and its variants see Carthery-Goulart[4]). EEP, as many other patients, was able to maintain an independent status, being able to work and drive for a long period after the onset of language symptoms. This was possible due to relative preservation of time and space orientation, episodic memory, and executive functions in the initial phase.

PPA-A is characterized by a progressive breakdown of syntactic processing and/or planning of motor speech (speech apraxia). In this variant, there is a gradual deterioration of the syntactic level of language, which is usually but not always accompanied by speech motor deficits. Those patients are nonfluent, that is, they present reduced verbal output and effortful, slow, and hesitant speech.[3]

In language production, PPA-A patients present at least one of the following two core characteristics: agrammatism (impairment in the production of grammatically correct sentences) and apraxia of speech (a disturbance in articulatory planning). Additionally, two out of three of the following features must be found: impaired comprehension of syntactically complex sentences, spared single-word comprehension, and spared object knowledge. As we see, EEP presented with all of these features. Regarding rate of speech, PPA-A patients present less than one-third the rate of elderly healthy individuals and these difficulties are usually more linked to grammatical processing deficits than to speech difficulties (apraxia of speech).[5]

Apraxia of speech is characterized by inconsistent speech sound errors (omissions, distortions, transpositions, insertions) and prosody changes. Patients and close relatives may notice those speech difficulties and refer to them as "stuttering" as in our case. Patients try to correct themselves, and hesitations and reformulations are common. For EEP, it seems that apraxia of speech was an important symptom for the reduction of oral output, as written production was more preserved than oral production. However, as oral communication is more time-constrained, it is possible that language difficulties were less pronounced when EEP was given more time for narrative production.

Comprehension of words, concepts, and simple sentences is spared in PPA-A. However, patients may display difficulties to process syntactically more complex sentences. EEP's sentence comprehension was more affected by grammatical complexity than by utterance length, as in other PPA-A patients, lending support to the syntactic nature of the deficits.

This clinical picture is different from the other two PPA variants. PPA-S starts with severe anomia and loss of word meanings, object, and people knowledge (a deficit affecting both verbal and nonverbal semantic memory in the course of the disease). PPA-L primarily affects phonological processing and verbal-auditory short-term memory in the absence of speech apraxia and frank agrammatism.[3]

Neuroimaging also differs in the three variants in the initial stage: PPA-A is related to predominant left posterior fronto-insular atrophy on MRI or predominant left posterior fronto-insular hypoperfusion or hypometabolism on SPECT or PET (as seen in EEP). PPA-S patients present with bilateral anterior temporal lobe atrophy, hypoperfusion, or hypometabolism usually greater in the left hemisphere and PPA-L predominantly shows atrophy in the left posterior temporo-parietal regions and predominant left posterior perisylvian or parietal hypoperfusion or hypometabolism.

EEP CSF findings must be interpreted with caution. There is no consensus regarding CSF biomarkers cutoff values among different centers; however, we state that the A-β 1-42 levels are marginally abnormal (low values), but tau and p-tau CSF levels are unequivocally normal (below most reported cutoff values). Recent longitudinal studies with serial clinical, CSF, and morphometric neuroimaging reanalysis[6] suggest that A-β 1-42 biomarker positivity in isolation is not sufficient to account for cognitive symptoms or brain atrophy, and may be present for many years in cognitively healthy subjects. Therefore, we argue that EEP had a neurodegenerative condition not associated with AD pathophysiology. Indeed, careful clinical characterization in combination with neuroimaging techniques that trace amyloid deposition in vivo show that PPA-A is usually not associated with AD.[7] Most of the case series with post-mortem pathological assessment were conducted before consensus diagnostic was established, in a recent era where logopenic and agrammatic variants were both regarded as nonfluent PPA. Although not ultimate, it seems that most of PPA-A cases, especially those that develop extrapyramidal syndromes, have an underlying pathology related to frontotemporal lobar degeneration with tau-positive inclusions.[8]

In the longitudinal course of the disease, as neurodegenerative disease spread out, these clinical profiles are less clear and symptoms of the different variants may co-occur. Other cognitive symptoms may also appear and pose more difficulties in everyday activities. In the described patient, the progression from mild stuttering to mutism occurred over 5 years but this rate of progression may vary significantly among cases. As said, PPA-A patients may also evolve with atypical parkinsonian syndromes (i.e., corticobasal syndrome and progressive supranuclear palsy) in later stages of the disease.

References

1. Machado TH, Campanha AC, Caramelli P, Carthery-Goulart MT. Brief intervention for agrammatism in Primary Progressive Nonfluent Aphasia: a case report. *Dement Neuropsychol.* 2014;8(3):291–296.

2. Mesulam MM. Primary progressive aphasia. *Ann. Neurol.* 2001;49:425–432.

3. Gorno-Tempini ML, Hillis AE, Weintraub S. Classification of primary progressive aphasia and its variants. *Neurology.* 2011;76:1006–1014.

4. Carthery-Goulart MT. Primary progressive aphasia. In: Pachana N (ed.) *Encyclopedia of Geropsychology.* Singapore, Springer Science+Business Media Singapore; 2016, pp. 1–11. doi: 10.1007/978-981-287-080-3_315-1.

5. Rascovsky K, Grossman M. Clinical diagnostic criteria and classification controversies in frontotemporal lobar degeneration. *Int. Rev. Psychiatry* 2013;25(2):145–158.

6. Sutphen CL, Jasielek MS, Shah AR, et al. Longitudinal cerebrospinal fluid biomarker changes in preclinical Alzheimer disease during middle age. *JAMA Neurol.* 2015;72:1029–1042.

7. Leyton CW, Villemagne VL, Savage S, et al. Subtypes of progressive aphasia: application of the International Consensus Criteria and validation using β-amyloid imaging. *Brain.* 2011;134:3030–3043.

8. Grossman M. The non-fluent/agrammatic variant of primary progressive aphasia. *Lancet Neurol.* 2012;11 (6):545–555.

Middle-Aged Man Looking for Words

Aline Carvalho Campanha, Mirna Lie Hosogi, Ricardo Nitrini, and Paulo Caramelli

16.1 Clinical History – Main Complaint

The patient is a 58-year-old-right-handed man, with 11 years of schooling. A retired bank manager, he presented in May 2011 with a 3-year history of progressive word-finding difficulties and phonological errors in spontaneous speech.

16.2 General History

According to the patient and his wife, he started to present with word-finding difficulties and changes in the sounds of words during speech in the last 3 years. His wife emphasized that his language alterations were the main symptoms for the initial phases of the disease. She observed that in the beginning he presented errors in spontaneous speech, could not finish sentences, and became progressively quieter and silent.

He avoided answering the phone and talking to his friends and relatives. At home, his family reported that besides the difficulties in verbal communication, he was no longer as emotive as he always had been. He was fully independent for daily life activities. During the last years working as a bank manager, he had to change function because of his communication difficulties, up to the point that he decided to retire.

16.3 Family History

The patient did not report any case of cognitive impairment or dementia in his family. His wife mentioned that he had slight learning disabilities during his childhood.

16.4 Assessment, Imaging and Test

The patient underwent the following tests:

16.4.1 Clinical Consultation and Neurological Examination

The present evaluation occurred 3 years before the beginning of the symptoms and was initially exclusive of language.

During the interview, the patient displayed several mistakes regarding personal facts, loss of objectivity, and difficulty in concentrating. His speech was marked by pauses and paraphasias, with naming difficulties. He had problems in keeping the contents of the conversation. Moreover, his wife reported difficulties to learn how to use home appliances and to express opinions verbally. Behavioral changes were also reported, such as anxiety, disinterest, social isolation, and lack of motivation. Sleep and appetite were preserved, although with preference for sweets. Delusions and hallucinations were absent.

Past medical history included only arterial hypertension. The patient was under regular drug treatment with hydrochlorothiazide (25 mg/day) and citalopram (20 mg/day).

On neurological examination, there were no motor or sensory deficits. Balance and gait were unremarkable. No signs of parkinsonian syndrome were detected. Cranial nerves were normal.

16.4.2 Cognitive and Functional Evaluations

The patient scored 21/30 in the Mini-Mental State Examination (MMSE); errors occurred in orientation to time/place, language, and memory tasks. He had difficulties in the clock-drawing test (Figure 16.1).

He scored 98/144 points in the Mattis Dementia Rating Scale (DRS). This score is below the Brazilian norms for the patient's educational level (i.e., 123/144). The patient displayed difficulties in almost all DRS domains: attention (32/37), initiative and perseveration (17/37), construction (6/6), concept (31/39), and memory (12/25). Episodic verbal memory was significantly impaired, with severe difficulty in immediate and delayed recall in the Rey Auditory-Verbal Learning Test (RAVLT).

Functional evaluation was conducted with the Disability Assessment for Dementia (DAD), with the following results: initiative (10/13 = 76%), planning and organization (8/10 = 80%), effective realization (13/17 = 76%), indicating mild functional impairment, essentially in instrumental activities of daily living dependent on oral communication.

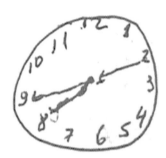

Figure 16.1 Patient's performance in the clock-drawing test (requested time – 2:45).

16.4.3 Speech and Language Assessment (Table 16.1)

- Spontaneous speech: The patient was fluent, but the speech was interrupted by pauses, word-finding problems, and phonemic errors, without phonoarticulatory distortions. The syntactic organization was preserved, without signs of agrammatism and without speech apraxia.
- Oral comprehension: Difficulties with comprehension of sentences, short texts and more complex syntactic constructions.
- Word repetition: Preserved from the Boston Diagnostic Aphasia Examination.
- Sentence repetition: Impaired with difficulties on repetition of phrases from the Boston Diagnostic Aphasia Examination.
- Naming: In the Boston naming test, he was able to name only 16 out of 60 items.
- Reading: The patient was able to read irregular and regular words, and also nonwords.
- Writing: He was able to write regular words and simple sentences.
- Buccofacial praxis: He was able to perform single and complex phonoarticulatory sequences.

16.4.4 Laboratory Tests and Neuroimaging Results

Magnetic resonance imaging (MRI) of the brain showed atrophy in the left hemisphere, particularly in the parietal lobe (Figure 16.2a and b).

Lumbar puncture was undertaken, with analysis of the cerebrospinal fluid-CSF (routine examination and investigation of Alzheimer's disease-AD biomarkers). Routine analysis was unremarkable. In the CSF, there was low concentration of beta-amyloid associated

Table 16.1 Patient's performance in language tests

Tasks Performance	
Oral comprehension	Score
Words (Cambridge test)	59/84
Orders (Boston)	9/14
Grammar interpretation	
Test for Reception of Grammar (TROG)	39/80
Repetition	
Words (Boston)	10/10
Repetition of sentences with high-frequency phrases (Boston)	4/10
Repetition of sentences with low-frequency phrases (Boston)	3/10
Confrontation naming	
Boston naming	16/60
Naming living things	12/32
Naming nonliving things	17/32
Semantic Fluency	
Animals	3
Fruits	4
Total	7
Faces – Recognition	14/15
Faces – Naming	9/15
Letter fluency	
F	5
A	4
S	7
Total	16
Camels and Cactus Test (CCT Cambridge Test)	40/64
Oral reading	
Words (Boston)	30/30
Sentences (Boston)	9/10
Writing	
Words (Boston)	30/30

Table 16.1 (cont.)

Sentences (Boston)	9/10
Semantic Definition	10/24
Praxis	Without phonoarticulatory problems

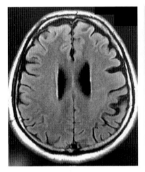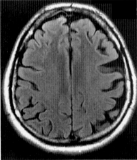

Figure 16.2 Axial T1 weighted MRI at ventricular level (a) and above the ventricles (b) showing enlarged sulci and cortical atrophy in the left hemisphere particularly in the parietal cortex

with high concentrations of tau and phospho-tau proteins, which are positive biomarkers of Alzheimer's disease.

16.5 Clinical and Etiological Diagnoses

The patient presented aphasia as the most prominent clinical feature and the main cause for impairment in daily life activities. Language deficits included anomia, poor word retrieval in spontaneous speech, difficulty in repeating sentences, and the presence of phonological errors. Structural (MRI) neuroimaging showed left hemisphere involvement, especially in temporal and parietal areas. Based on these clinical and imaging findings and in accordance with the criteria proposed by Gorno-Tempini et al.,[1] the patient was diagnosed with primary progressive aphasia (PPA), logopenic subtype (lvPPA). Positivity of the three CSF AD biomarkers indicates the diagnosis of AD.

16.6 Discussion

Although the patient has only sought treatment after 3 years since the beginning of symptoms, the first complaints were related exclusively to difficulties in oral communication.

PPA is diagnosed when language impairment arises in relative isolation and progresses to become the primary obstacle to daily functioning. Frontotemporal lobar degeneration and AD are the most common neuropathological diagnoses.[2] A 2011 diagnosis consensus[1] described recommendations for recognizing three common forms and use of parameters for classification of variants. Each variant has specific linguistic characteristics and they are essential for PPA subtype classification: nonfluent/agrammatic, semantic, and logopenic.

With respect to oral language we could observe that the patient was fluent, but the speech was interrupted by pauses, word-finding problems and phonemic errors, without speech apraxia and agrammatism (Table 16.1). The pauses present in spontaneous speech in the logopenic variant of PPA are characterized by slow rate and are distinct from those found in patients with nonfluent PPA that are marked by motor speech errors and agrammatism.

Although naming problems are present in the other PPA subtypes, in the semantic variant, naming impairment is more severe and occurs in conjunction with marked difficulties in single word comprehension. Moreover, semantic memory impairment causes difficulties in object and face recognition. On the other hand, in the logopenic variant of PPA the naming errors are usually phonologic in nature and not due to semantic memory problems. Naming impairment is usually less severe in logopenic than in semantic variant.

Repetition of sentences is impaired in logopenic PPA. Phonologic short-term memory deficit is a key cognitive mechanism underlying most language deficits in this PPA variant. Comprehension of long sentences might be compromised, probably due to limitations in auditory working memory.[3] The sentence comprehension is more influenced by length and word frequency than by grammatical complexity.[1] Accordingly, the repetition of single words can be spared.

As we know, language is a complex activity that depends on the integrity of other functions to be performed in a satisfactory manner, such as the phonological loop of working memory.

Although semantic memory impairment is not evident in logopenic PPA, the patient had difficulties in semantic definitions and oral comprehension. He failed when he had to understand words or orders presented orally and to interpret different grammatically sentences. Sentence comprehension can also be impaired in logopenic variants and this finding may be related to sentence length and to difficulties in keeping the sentence in the working memory system during decoding of the verbal material.

We can suggest that the patient's performance on neuropsychological tests may have suffered interference from his language disorder, as it happened in verbal episodic memory assessment (RAVLT). Cognitive differences have been identified in individuals with PPA compared to other neurodegenerative disorders, such as frontotemporal dementia and typical AD, and are particularly evident on measures of language, verbal memory, and attention. Moreover, patients with logopenic PPA perform poorly on most neurocognitive impairment when compared with other PPA variants that reflect compromise to different brain regions or circuitry.[4]

Although the clinical syndrome of logopenic aphasias is commonly associated with AD pathology, the presentation and clinical course, as well as the pattern of cognitive deficits, argue against a typical presentation of AD. The distinction between logopenic variant and dementia with prominent language involvement may be difficult to establish in some cases.

Atrophy in the left hemisphere seen on MRI, particularly in the parietal lobe (Figure 16.2a and b), supports the diagnosis of logopenic variant of PPA. The combination of low beta-amyloid, and increased total tau and phosphorylated tau proteins on CSF confirms the etiological diagnosis of AD, the most common underlying pathology found in logopenic PPA.

References

1. Gorno-Tempini ML, Hillis AE, Weintraub S, et al. Classification of primary progressive aphasia and its variants. *Neurology*. 2011;76:1006–1014.

2. Rogalski E, Sridhar J, Rader B, et al. Aphasic variant of Alzheimer disease: clinical, anatomic and genetic features. *Neurology*. 2016;87: 1337–1343.

3. Mesulam MM, Rogalski EJ, Wieneke C, et al. Primary progressive aphasia and the evolving neurology of the language network. *Nat Rev Neurol*. 2014;10: 554–569.

4. Butts AM, Machulda MM, Duffy JR, et al. Neuropsychological profiles differ among the three variants of Primary Progressive Aphasia. *J Int Neuropsychol Soc*. 2015;21:429–435.

The Man Who Stopped Reading

William S. Musser, Julia Kofler, James T. Becker, and Oscar L. Lopez

17.1 Clinical History – Chief Complaint

This is about a 56-year-old man who presented to the neurology clinic because of reading difficulty.

17.2 General History

Five years before the evaluation, the patient's wife noted that he became "forgetful" and would require gentle prompting to complete tasks. She also noticed that he had "lost interest" in reading. Bilateral cataracts were found on ophthalmologic examination but their removal did not improve his reading.

At the time of evaluation in the cognitive disorders clinic, the patient reported difficulty with reading. He described knowing the letters of the alphabet but said that "I have difficulty putting them together." He said that he could not follow written instructions, but had no difficulty with writing. Other cognitive symptoms were present as well. He would begin familiar tasks at home (i.e., walking the dog, mowing the lawn, taking out the trash) but could not complete them without verbal cueing. He had difficulty following multistep commands. He could no longer set the table for dinner. Nevertheless, he still managed the family's checkbook, paying bills without making errors. He continued to drive but required others in the car to read street signs for him. However, he was still able to identify symbols on traffic signs. His family reported that he had become sedentary and lacked motivation. His attention to personal hygiene was mostly preserved but he had stopped brushing his teeth regularly. An 8-month trial of donepezil 10 mg at bedtime produced no benefit.

17.3 Family History

His daughter was diagnosed with dyslexia. There was no history of dementia or neurodegenerative disorder in the immediate family.

17.4 Examination

The patient had a detailed clinical exam at the Alzheimer's Disease Research Center at the University of Pittsburgh.[1] His initial score on the Folstein Mini-Mental State Examination (MMSE) was 27/30.[2] He was oriented to person only. He correctly calculated the number of quarters in $6.75 (but he thought that his answer was incorrect). He named the months of the year in reverse order correctly. He had rare phonemic paraphasic errors and could not read written text when presented to him but he could identify the individual letters. There was no ideational or ideomotor apraxia, or neglect. Stereognosis was intact but he had mild agraphesthesia on the right side. No frontal release signs were noted.

Blood tests and chemistries were normal. The MRI of the brain showed mild left temporal lobe atrophy. A SPECT scan at the time of initial evaluation showed bilateral parietal hypoperfusion, left worse than right.

17.5 Diagnosis

The initial diagnosis was non-Alzheimer's dementia/partial angular gyrus syndrome with alexia without agraphia.

17.6 Follow-Up

One year later, the MMSE score was 22/30. The alexia had worsened. He could no longer read labels (his family described his misidentifying a can of black spray paint as "wasp spray"). He could not find a particular object in a group of objects (i.e., locate a box of garbage bags in a full pantry). He had started to make financial errors with his checkbook. On exam, color agnosia and phonemic paraphasias were present as were a right palmomental and snout reflex.

Two years later, the MMSE was 21/30. Word-finding difficulties and color agnosia persisted. In addition, he tended to forget portions of conversations, and developed obsessive ideas and perseverative behaviors. He preferred to wear the same set of clothes each day. He assisted with drying dishes but could not place them in the correct cupboard. On exam, he could not read a sentence but was able to compose a simple one.

Three years after his initial evaluation, the MMSE was 20/30, and it continued to decline over the ensuing 2 years. A graph of the annual MMSE scores is

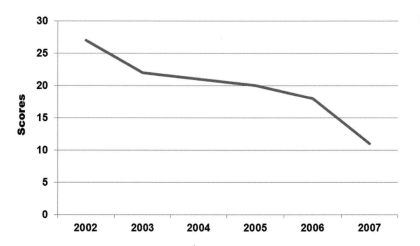

Figure 17.1 The Mini-Mental State Examination scores during follow-up.

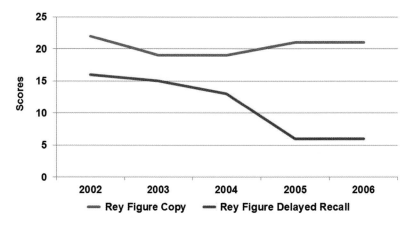

Figure 17.2 The copy and delayed recall of the modified Rey-Osterrieth figure.

shown in Figure 17.1. A graph with his scores on the modified Rey-Osterrieth Figure Copy scores is shown in Figure 17.2,[3] demonstrating preservation of the copying skills with a decline in drawing the diagram from memory.

During his last clinical examination, it was noted that he could no longer pick out clothes from his closet. He could not identify the family car. He could not identify relatives by name and was unable to recognize his own daughter. He misidentified objects (i.e., a bag of potato chips for a coffee cup, an apple for an orange). He repeated himself. On exam, he could not state his date of birth nor his age. He could not calculate the number of quarters in a dollar amount (e.g., $6.75). He could not add a pair of two-digit numbers. He could not read the word "CAT." He could not transcribe a four-word sentence. He could not identify objects (i.e., a cotton ball or

piece of aluminum foil) by either sight or feel. His diagnosis was changed to probable Alzheimer's disease with an atypical presentation.[4] He died at the age of 69, 18 years after the onset of the symptoms, and 12 years after his initial evaluation.

17.7 Autopsy

Gross examination of the brain revealed lobar atrophy of frontal and temporal lobes with extension into inferior parietal lobe but relative preservation of pre/postcentral gyri. The atrophy was asymmetric with more severe changes seen on the left side. Microscopic examination found severe neuronal loss and gliosis in the anterior mesial temporal cortex, insular cortex, mid-frontal, temporal cortex, and inferior parietal cortex. Numerous Pick bodies were seen throughout most of the cortex (Figure 17.3), mixed with pre-

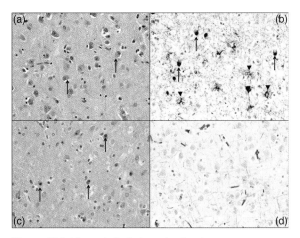

Figure 17.3 Histopathological examination demonstrates numerous round basophilic inclusions on hematoxylin & eosin stained tissue sections (panel A). These Pick bodies are highlighted by immunohistochemical stains for phospho-tau (PHF1; panel B) and 3-repeat tau (RD3; panel C), but are negative on a Gallyas silver stain which only labels 4-repeat tau aggregates (panel D). PHF1 stains also highlight numerous neuropil threads and ramified astrocytes. [400× all images; arrows indicate Pick bodies; arrowheads indicate ramified astrocytes].

tangles, neuropil threads, and glial tau pathology in the form of ramified astrocytes and oligodendroglial coiled bodies. No amyloid deposition was found. Moderate atherosclerotic and mild arteriolosclerotic changes were seen. The final neuropathological diagnosis was Pick's disease.

17.8 Discussion

The determination of the neuropathological basis of dementing disorders based on clinical data can be difficult in cases with unusual signs and symptoms, especially in younger individuals (e.g., 60 years old). In addition while clinicians expect to identify clearly defined clinical entities, there can be both significant overlap between syndromes and a blurring of the boundaries between syndromes often occurs as the dementia progresses.

Frontotemporal degeneration (FTD) is a term used to include a group of non-Alzheimer dementias, whose pathological basis includes focal neuronal loss and gliosis in the frontal and temporal lobes lobes.[5,6] In approximately 70% of the patients the symptoms start before age 65, and the prevalence ranges from 1 to 26/100,000,000.[7] Clinically, patients with FTD can present a variety of syndromes including behavioral symptoms (the behavioral variant of FTD), primary progressive aphasia,[8] semantic dementia,[9,10]

cortico-basal degeneration,[11] progressive supranuclear palsy,[12] or motor neuron disease,[13] or a combination of one or more syndromes.[11] Pathologically, FTD is associated with deposition of tau, TAR DNA-binding protein 43 (TDP-43), and fused in sarcoma (*fus*) proteins,[14–16] although FTD-tau accounts for >50% of the cases.[17]

Pick's disease is a rare form of FTD first described by Arnold Pick in 1892.[18] It accounts for <5% of the autopsy series of dementias[19] and 30% of the FTD cases.[17] It affects both men and women, and tends to progress faster than Alzheimer's disease (AD).[20] The clinical symptoms usually involve abnormal behavior (e.g., disinhibition, impulsiveness),[21] language disorders,[22] or both, consistent with frontotemporal lobe dysfunction, as occurs with other non-Pick's disease FTD cases. However, the clinical presentation and progression of the symptoms is not uniform,[23] and there are case reports with a predominantly apraxic syndrome that mimicked cortico-basal degeneration with an asymmetric involvement of the parietal lobes.[24,25] The most important neuropathological lesion is the presence of neuronal loss, gliosis, and round intraneuronal inclusions called "Pick's bodies," which are composed of tau proteins enriched with 3-repeat isoforms. Pick's disease predominantly affects the limbic, paralimbic, and neocortical regions, and can extend to primary motor and visual regions, basal ganglia, cerebellum, and midbrain structures in more advanced stages.[26] Because of the involvement of the mesial temporal lobe structures (e.g., dentate gyrus of the hippocampus), some cases can present with memory loss indistinguishable from AD.[27,28]

Because the initial findings in this patient involved most prominently a loss of reading ability with a focal hypoperfusion of the parietal lobes, the initial diagnostic formulation for this patient was a neurodegenerative process involving the dominant inferior parietal lobe with components of the angular gyrus syndrome rather than AD. The angular gyrus syndrome includes alexia with agraphia, fluent aphasia, visuoconstructional deficits, and Gerstmann's syndrome (i.e., acalculia, agraphia, right/left disorientation, and finger agnosia).[29,30] Reasoning was relatively preserved at baseline, but deteriorated over time,[31] and no episodes of abnormal behavior (e.g., disinhibition, agitation, inappropriate behavior) were reported. The incomplete syndrome seen here represents a heterogeneous involvement of the inferior parietal lobes, and suggests that the disease process may have not started in the typical frontal-temporal lobe areas, as expected.[32] The determinants of this unusual initial pathological involvement are not well understood and are difficult to examine when the disease has been present for several years, and the pathology is widely distributed at the time of the autopsy. However, the asymmetric involvement of the parietal lobes has been shown in patients with Pick's disease whose initial presentation mimicked a cortico-basal degeneration syndrome.[24,25]

Alexia without agraphia, the loss of reading ability but with sparing of the ability to write, also known as pure alexia, is due to a disconnection between visual input and language areas of the brain.[33] The usual causes are lesions affecting the left calcarine cortex and the splenium of the corpus callosum.[34] Because of the distribution of the neurodegenerative process, the most likely explanation in our case is (a) a cortical deficit beginning in the parietal lobes, or (b) a cortical-cortical disconnection affecting the occipital inputs to the parietal lobes, or (c) both, which may also explain his color agnosia.[35] Interestingly, there are familial FTD cases whose initial symptom was agraphia.[36] However, it was difficult to determine whether that agraphia was part of a true aphasic syndrome, or it was related to a dysexecutive, apraxic, or visuoconstructive deficit. Nevertheless, these patients showed a frontotemporal lobe pattern of impairment in functional neuroimaging studies and had a more widespread language deficit.

Although the most salient initial symptom was alexia without agraphia, this patient also had a short-term memory loss. Over the first 5 years following his diagnosis, these deficits progressed and new cognitive-behavioral difficulties developed. These new symptoms involved practically all cognitive domains, especially those ascribed to the frontal and temporal lobes, as well as to the inferior parietal cortex. Importantly, his visuoconstructional functions remained relatively stable during the follow-up time, which is consistent with the relative sparing of the superior parietal lobe regions found at autopsy. In addition, he developed memory loss, nonfluent aphasia with significant semantic errors, impaired semantic knowledge, and deficits in planning and multitasking. This prompted a change in his clinical diagnosis from a non-AD dementia to an atypical presentation of AD. At autopsy 5 years later the sole neuropathological diagnosis was Pick's disease.

The patient presented with language dysfunction in the form of alexia, and mild behavioral change, but that change was limited to a subtle lack of motivation and adoption of a sedentary lifestyle. As his cognitive difficulties progressed, so did his behavioral dysfunction. However, his cognitive difficulties were more noticeable to the patient and his family. His language dysfunction was very prominent, progressive, and easily quantifiable. This combination of factors led to the incorrect clinical diagnosis. Even with the clinical skills present in today's cognitive neurology clinics, the clinical diagnosis of an unusual subtype of dementia can be incorrect. The use of biomarkers for amyloid deposition,[37] or tau proteins[38] will help to improve clinical diagnosis in these type of patients.

Acknowledgments

This chapter was supported, in part, by grants P50-AG005133, R01-AG20098, and UF1-AG051197 from National Institute on Aging.

References

1. Lopez OL, Becker JT, Klunk W, et al. Research evaluation and diagnosis of probable Alzheimer's disease over the last two decades: I. *Neurology*. 2000;55 (12):1854–1862.

2. Folstein MF, Folstein SE, McHugh, PR. Mini-mental state: a practical method grading the cognitive state of patients for the clinician. *Psychiatr Res*. 1975;12:189–198.

3. Saxton JA, Becker JT, Wisniewski S. The ROCF and dementia. In: Knight JA, ed. *The Handbook of Rey-Osterrieth Complex Figure Usage: Clinical and Research Applications*. Lutz, FL: Psychological Assessment Resources, Inc.; 2003: 569–582.

4. McKhann G, Drachman D, Folstein M, et al. Clinical diagnosis of Alzheimer's disease: report of the NINCDS-ADRDA Work Group under the auspices of Department of Health and Human Services Task Force on Alzheimer's Disease. *Neurology*. 1984;34(7):939–944.

5. McKhann GM, Albert MS, Grossman M, et al. Clinical and pathological diagnosis of frontotemporal dementia. *Arch Neurol*. 2001;58: 1803–1809.

6. Neary D, Snowden JS, Gustafson L, et al. Frontotemporal lobar degeneration: a consensus on

clinical diagnostic criteria. *Neurology.* 1998;51(6):1546–1554.

7. Knopman DS, Roberts RO. Estimating the number of persons with frontotemporal lobar degeneration in the US population. *J Mol Neurosci.* 2011;45(3):330–335.

8. Mesulam MM. Primary progressive aphasia. *Ann Neurol.* 2001;49(4):425–432.

9. Hodges JR, Patterson K, Oxbury S, Funnell E. Semantic dementia: progressive fluent aphasia with temporal lobe atrophy. *Brain.* 1992;115:1783–1806.

10. Mesulam M, Rogalski E, Wieneke C, et al. Neurology of anomia in the semantic variant of primary progressive aphasia. *Brain.* 2009;132(Pt 9):2553–2565.

11. Josephs KA, Petersen RC, Knopman DS, et al. Clinicopathologic analysis of frontotemporal and corticobasal degenerations and PSP. *Neurology.* 2006;66(1): 41–48.

12. Respondek G, Stamelou M, Kurz C, et al. The phenotypic spectrum of progressive supranuclear palsy: a retrospective multicenter study of 100 definite cases. *Mov Disord.* 2014;29(14):1758–1766.

13. Burrell JR, Halliday GM, Kril JJ, et al. The frontotemporal dementia-motor neuron disease continuum. *Lancet.* 2016;388 (10047):919–931.

14. Mackenzie IR, Ansorge O, Strong M, et al. Pathological heterogeneity in amyotrophic lateral sclerosis with FUS mutations: two distinct patterns correlating with disease severity and mutation. *Acta Neuropathol.* 2011;**122**(1):87–98.

15. Mackenzie IR, Baker M, Pickering-Brown S, et al. The neuropathology of frontotemporal lobar degeneration caused by mutations in the progranulin gene. *Brain.* 2006;129 (Pt 11):3081–3090.

16. Tan RH, Kril JJ, Fatima M, et al. TDP-43 proteinopathies: pathological identification of brain regions differentiating clinical phenotypes. *Brain.* 2015;138:3110–3122.

17. Bang J, Spina S, Miller BL. Frontotemporal dementia. *Lancet.* 2015;386(10004):1672–1682.

18. Pick A. Ueber primäre chronische Demenz (so. Dementia praecox) im jugendlichen Alter. *Prager Med Wochenschr.* 1891;16:312–315.

19. Barker WW, Luis CA, Kashuba A, et al. Relative frequencies of Alzheimer disease, Lewy body, vascular and frontotemporal dementia, and hippocampal sclerosis in the State of Florida Brain Bank. *Alzheimer Dis Assoc Disord.* 2002;16(4):203–212.

20. Kertesz A. Clinical features and diagnosis of frontotemporal dementia. *Front Neurol Neurosci.* 2009;24:140–148.

21. Constantinidis J. Pick dementia: Anatamoclinical correlations and pathophysiological considerations. *Interdiscipl Topics Geront.* 1985;19:72–97.

22. Graff-Radford NR, Damasio AR, Hyman BT, et al. Progressive aphasia in a patient with Pick's disease: a neuropsychological, radiologic, and anatomic study. *Neurology.* 1990;40:620–626.

23. Piguet O, Halliday GM, Reid WG, et al. Clinical phenotypes in autopsy-confirmed Pick disease. *Neurology.* 2011;76(3):253–259.

24. Cambier J, Masson M, Dairou R, Henin D. Etude anatomo-clinique d'une forme pariétale de maladie de Pick. *Rev Neurol (Paris).* 1981;137:33–38.

25. Lang AE, Bergeron C, Pollanen MS, Ashby P, et al. Parietal Pick's disease mimicking cortical-basal ganglionic degeneration. *Neurology.* 1994;44 (8):1436–1440.

26. Irwin DJ, Brettschneider J, McMillan CT, et al. Deep clinical

and neuropathological phenotyping of Pick disease. *Ann Neurol.* 2016;79(2):272–287. doi: 10.1002/ana.24559.

27. Armstrong RA, Cairns NJ, Lantos PL. Clustering of Pick bodies in patients with Pick's disease. *Neurosci Lett.* 1998;242(2): 81–84.

28. Dickson DW, Kouri N, Murray ME, Josephs KA. Neuropathology of frontotemporal lobar degeneration-tau (FTLD-tau). *J Mol Neurosci.* 2011;45 (3):384–389.

29. Benson DF, Cummings JL, Tsai SY. Angular gyrus syndrome simulating Alzheimer's disease. *Arch Neurol.* 1982;39:616–620.

30. Eidelberg D, Galaburda, AM. Inferior parietal lobule. Divergent architectonic asymmetries in the human brain. *Arch Neurol.* 1984;41(8):843–852.

31. Wicklund AH, Johnson N, Weintraub S. Preservation of reasoning in primary progressive aphasia: further differentiation from Alzheimer's disease and the behavioral presentation of frontotemporal dementia. *J Clin Exp Neuropsychol.* 2004;26 (3):347–355.

32. Irwin DJ, Grossman M, Weintraub D, et al. Neuropathological and genetic correlates of survival and dementia onset in synucleinopathies: a retrospective analysis. *Lancet Neurol.* 2017;16 (1):55–65.

33. Geschwind N. Disconnexion syndromes in animals and man. *Brain.* 1965;88:237–294.

34. Damasio AR, Damasio H. The anatomic basis of pure alexia. *Neurology.* 1983;33:1573–1583.

35. Geschwind N, Fusillo M. Color-naming defects in association with alexia. *Arch Neurol.* 1966;15 (2):137–146.

36. Sitek EJ, Narozanska E, Barczak A, et al. Agraphia in patients with frontotemporal dementia and

parkinsonism linked to
chromosome 17 with P301L
MAPT mutation: dysexecutive,
aphasic, apraxic or spatial
phenomenon? *Neurocase.* 2014;
20(1):69–86.

37. Klunk WE, Engler H, Nordberg A,
et al. Imaging brain amyloid
in Alzheimer's disease with
Pittsburgh Compound-B.
Ann Neurol. 2004;55:
306–319.

38. Johnson KA, Schultz A,
Betensky RA, et al. Tau positron
emission tomographic imaging
in aging and early Alzheimer
disease. *Ann Neurol.* 2016;
79(1):110–119.

A Meaningless World

Paolo Vitali and Simona Maria Brambati

A 54-year-old right-handed highly educated French-speaking father of three was referred for a neuro-logical consultation for "some memory difficulties and behavioral changes" for the past 2 years. His past medical history was unremarkable and no learning disabilities were reported. He denied alcohol and drug abuse and he did not smoke. His father and two of his paternal aunts had been diagnosed with late-onset Alzheimer's disease. He was concerned by the possibility of being affected by the same neurodegenerative condition.

He reported increasing difficulties in remembering names, such as object and proper names, popular films, or familiar places, for example, the names of the ski trails at the resort where he had worked for a long time as an associate director. He was recently forced to quit his job, one of the reasons being that he seemed unable to understand what his colleagues were saying. Moreover, he forgot the meaning of the items on his shopping list and he needed pictures to pick up the right items at the grocery store. He also reported new difficulties in recognizing people and often questioned whether he had already met the person that was in front of him. He began to forget how to cook and had to be supervised when trying to remember previously known recipes and procedures. He became more confused concerning arithmetical facts and had difficulty understanding and distinguishing numbers (e.g., 200 – 2,000 – 200,000) and with orthography (word spelling). He occasionally had trouble paying attention to his interlocutor because he was focused on trying to remember the appropriate word to say, and the family also noted difficulty with word comprehension as well as with following group conversations. Sometimes he appeared "absent" and indifferent. He needed more encouragement with respect to activities of daily living (cooking, shopping, going out, etc.). However, he was still able to problem solve and fix things, like changing a bicycle wheel, for example. He also continued to be physically active and went to ski regularly.

He tried to cope with his progressive difficulties by keeping a diary in which he noted several specific items belonging to different general categories (e.g., furniture, fruits, vegetables, etc.) as a tool to be referred to in case of a forgotten name. He could remember that the specific item he was looking for was on the list and could find it among others. Nevertheless, he admitted that sometimes he put an item on the list and then forgot what it was for. He also tried to retrieve words by adopting a self-cueing phonological strategy. In fact, sometimes he could remember the first syllable of the word, which was then used as a cue to enhance access to the lexical target. However, he found irregular French words challenging.

On examination, his oral spontaneous expressive language was fluent with a speech rate that was generally high, well-articulated, and grammatically appropriate. However, his speech quality was mildly reduced due to word-finding difficulties (anomia). Although rare, he produced syllable substitutions when generating less frequent words, which resulted in occasional pseudo-words (phonological paraphasia). Oral comprehension was adequate in a familiar environment. Yet, more complex explanations were difficult to follow. The remainder of his neurological examination was normal, including the absence of frontal release signs, parkinsonism, or alien-limb phenomenon.

On further cognitive testing (Table 18.1), he scored 23 out of 30 on the Montreal Cognitive Assessment (MoCA). Executive functions and visuospatial abilities were well preserved. Working memory was only mildly impaired. An apparent dissociation was observed between a preserved visuospatial episodic memory – the delayed recall of the Rey Complex Figure – and an impaired verbal episodic memory. The latter was assessed using a list of 16 words to remember across 3 learning series. Despite a defective performance on free and cued recall and an absence of a learning curve after the 3 repetitions, delayed word recognition was within the normal range with 14 out of 16 correct recognitions and no false intrusions. This finding argues against the hypothesis of an impaired storage mechanism for verbal material in this patient, as usually observed in classic amnestic dementia (e.g., Alzheimer's disease).

Extensive speech-language evaluation (Table 18.1) showed severe picture-naming impairment – even for high-frequency items – along with deficits in object recognition. Semantic and phonological verbal

Table 18.1 Neuropsychological and language profiles of svPPA patient

Tests	Scores
Cognitive general functioning	
MoCA	23[a]
Vocabulary (WAIS)	23[a]
Information (WAIS)	8[a]
Executive functions	
Trail Making Test – A (s)/B (s)	27/76
Working memory	
Digit span – forward/backward	4[a]/3[a]
Visuo-spatial ability	
Complex Rey Figure – Copy	
Score/Time (s)	34/224
Episodic memory	
Complex Rey Figure	
Immediate recall: Score/Time (s)	25.5/63
Delayed recall: Score/Time (s)	21.5/55
Gröber and Buschke 16 words	
Immediate recall	15
Free recall 1	6[a]
Free recall 2	4[a]
Free recall 3	4[a]
Total recall	15[a]
Delayed free recall	3[a]
Total delayed recall	3[a]
Recognition – true	14
Recognition – false	0
Language	
Verbal fluency (90 s)	
Phonemic (P)	8[a]
Semantic (animals)	6[a]
Picture Naming	
Boston Naming Test (/60)	5[a]
Explicit semantics	
Pyramid and Palm Tree Test words (/56)	26[a]
pictures (/52)	37[a]
Word-to-picture matching: "Repeat and Point test" (/10)	7[a]
Mill Hill Synonymous judgment (/34)	11[a]
Oral Verbal comprehension	
Single word comprehension (Lexis) (/64)	48[a]
Sentence comprehension (MT86)	Normal
Written syntactic comprehension	
Chapman-Cook Test	2[a]
Oral Repetition	
ODEDYS Word Repetition Test (/16)	16
ODEDYS Pseudo-Word Repetition Test (/20)	18

[a] Defective performance based on published norms.

fluency were also drastically reduced. Reading of regular words was intact, whereas he had difficulty reading pseudo-words and irregular words (surface dyslexia). Oral repetition was adequate. Interestingly, single-word oral comprehension was severely impaired while sentence comprehension was better (despite mild difficulties with the passive voice) suggesting a facilitating effect from the context on disrupted semantics. Reading comprehension was similarly impaired, but he could benefit from re-reading the text. Written expression was reduced, slow, and simplified, and some graphemic paragraphias and grammatical error agreements were observed (surface dysorthography) (Figure 18.1). Explicit semantics was clearly impaired as assessed by several tests based on semantic processing of words and pictures (semantic matching). For example, he was no more able to process the relationship between *owl* (a nocturnal bird) and *night*.

Subsequent language evaluations revealed an increased number of anomias and circumlocutions in spontaneous speech, and deteriorated picture naming with loss of benefit from phonological cueing. Speech became more laborious and tangential. He also developed new difficulties concerning the pragmatic aspects of language, misunderstanding interlocutor's intentions and not respecting tour-de-role in conversations. Monologues became easier for him than dialogues.

A visual review of his 3-Tesla brain MRI demonstrated severe left anterior temporal lobe (ATL)

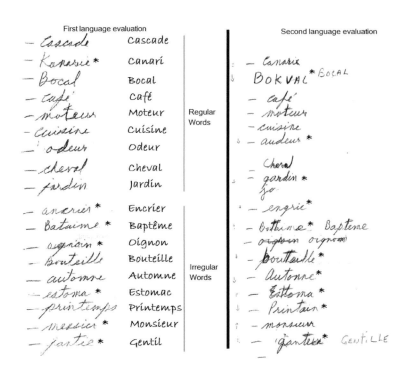

First language evaluation | Second language evaluation

Regular Words:

	Cascade
	Canari *
	Bocal
	Café
	Moteur
	Cuisine
	Odeur
	Cheval
	Jardin

Irregular Words:

	Encrier *
	Baptême *
	Oignon *
	Bouteille
	Automne
	Estomac *
	Printemps
	Monsieur *
	Gentil *

Figure 18.1 Examples of French irregular misspelled words (identified by the * in the figure) in two subsequent svPPA patient's language evaluations. Note the occurrence even of regular misspelled words as the disease progresses.

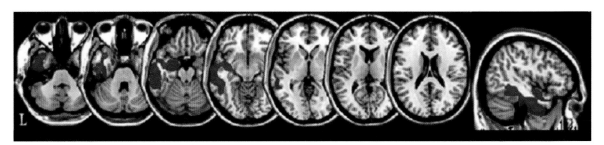

Figure 18.2 Pattern of gray matter atrophy in the svPPA patient compared to 18 age- and sex-matched healthy controls using VBM as implemented in spm8 software.

atrophy and moderate atrophy of the right temporal pole, with relative sparing of the mesial temporal regions. This characteristic pattern of gray matter atrophy was subsequently quantified by using a Voxel-Based Morphometry (VBM) analysis (Figure 18.2). Based on his language profile and neuroimaging findings, a diagnosis of imaging-supported semantic-variant Primary Progressive Aphasia (svPPA) was made.

PPA is a neurodegenerative condition character-ized by insidious onset and gradual progression of relatively isolated language difficulties (aphasia) for the first 2 years of the disease. Age of symptom onset is generally between 50 and 70 and life expectancy is 14 years, which is longer than in AD. Typically,

episodic memory and visuospatial systems remain relatively preserved in the first years of the disease. This often helps patients preserve autonomy in most activities of daily living for a long time (e.g., self-care), except those related to communication (e.g., using a phone). However, the impact of language deficits on communication abilities has a devastating effect on both social and work life with a major impact on patients' and caregivers' quality of life. The language domain continues to be disproportionally impaired even after the target of neurodegeneration has pro-gressed from the peak-atrophy site in the language-dominant hemisphere to involve other cognitive domains. Depending on which language system is defective, three clinical PPA variants (nonfluent/

agrammatic, semantic, and logopenic) have been clinically and anatomically well characterized in the literature. In the present chapter, we are focusing on the svPPA. The svPPA, also known as temporal variant Fronto-Temporal Dementia (FTD) or semantic dementia (SD), is defined by isolated semantic deficits which result in both expressive (word finding or object naming) and receptive (single-word comprehension) language impairments. The diagnostic criteria for this syndrome were first published by Neary et al. in 1998, but more recent diagnostic criteria have been established by an international expert consensus in 2011.[1] As clearly observed in our patient, the core feature of the disease is the loss of word meaning, especially for low-frequency and low-familiarity items. This reflects the more general loss of knowledge concerning objects (as per the diagnostic criteria), as well as public facts, known people, and concepts (e.g., "religion") stored in a disrupted semantic system. Difficulties in reading and spelling irregular words (surface dyslexia and surface dysorthography) also reflect an impaired semantic system and represent critical features of the disease in accord to published diagnostic criteria. On the other hand, oral repetition and speech production (grammar and motor speech) must be preserved.

Per one of the most prominent cognitive models of the anterior temporal region's function, these bilateral structures would support conceptual knowledge, combining information from sensory-, motor- and language-specific areas.[2] Not surprisingly, svPPA is radiologically characterized by striking atrophy (or hypoperfusion/hypometabolism on SPECT or PET scans) of anterior temporal regions. While this brain atrophy is often asymmetrical early in the disease (with the left regions usually being more involved), it becomes more symmetrical with the progression of the disease.[3] The spreading of atrophy to the right ATL is usually associated with behavioral changes, such as a decline in empathy and the emergence of coldness in personality profiles, increased rigidity, obsessive behaviors, and interrupting others, like our patient.

The presence of semantic memory deficits in this patient has been proven by a series of experimental semantic tasks.[4] In a famous face-naming task, he was not able to correctly name any single famous people, while healthy subjects correctly named 75% of the presented celebrities. When he was asked to match a verbally presented proper name with the corresponding face in an array of four black-and-white pictures, which comprised three famous people and an unknown distracter (famous-proper-name-to-face matching task), and to specify the profession of the famous person and provide some biographical details about the target (semantic categorization based on profession), the svPPA patient – even at the early stages of the disease – showed extremely low performance in both famous-proper-name-to-face matching (accuracy = 38.5%, performance 10 SD below the mean of the control group) and semantic categorization (accuracy = 30.8%, performance 38 SD below the mean of the control group) tests. These results suggest that his difficulties with famous face naming reflect person-related semantic deficits. This was confirmed by using a semantic priming paradigm, which does not require explicit access to lexical and semantic information. The expression "semantic priming effect" refers to the facilitation in stimulus processing induced by the prior presentation of a semantically associated stimulus. Specifically, it has been shown that in healthy controls, it takes less time to decide whether a target proper name belongs to a famous person when it is preceded by the name of a famous person sharing the same profession (prime word) (e.g., "Marlon Brando-Paul Newman"). Cognitive models on the organization of the semantic system explain this effect as resulting from automatic spreading of the activation of the semantic network from the node represented by the prime word to the node represented by the target word. Therefore, this effect is expected to be absent or reduced in patients with degraded person-specific semantic information. Accordingly, the svPPA patient showed no facilitation effects in the semantic priming task. On the contrary, the familiarity judgment task was slowed when the target famous name was preceded by a prime sharing the same profession.

The distinguishing dissociation between preserved episodic memory and impaired semantic memory in svPPA could explain an interesting clinical observation in these patients. They usually manifest intact memory of recent autobiographical life events and disproportional forgetfulness of remote events that have lost self-centered features and have become "semantics". This memory profile is exactly the opposite of that observed in classic mnestic syndromes, where the hippocampus-depending anterograde episodic memory functioning is defective. This prevents the storage of new information in the memory system, while the ancient, well-consolidated mnestic traces are not lost (a phenomenon known as the Ribot law of episodic memory). In svPPA, on the contrary, the preservation of the episodic autobiographical memory system helps recalling specifically self-interested details concerning objects, peoples, or facts. On the other hand, collectively shared knowledge – deprived of ego-referential features – is semantics, and thus more fragile and prone to be forgotten.

svPPA is most often linked to TDP43-positive neuronal (cytoplasmic) inclusions type C pathology, in contrast with other neurodegenerative conditions belonging to the FTD clinical spectrum, where the clinicopathological correlation is more heterogeneous. TDP43 is an RNA- and DNA-binding protein that is normally found mainly in the nucleus where it is believed to regulate gene expression. In accord to recent evidences,[5] TDP43 likely contributes directly to the disease through its mislocalization to an unexpected place – the mitochondria – where it prevents assembly of part of the respiratory chain. However, histopathologic evidences of other neurodegenerative pathologies (e.g., tau, Pick, AD) have been occasionally observed in svPPA. Familial cases of svPPA are very rare, even if an autosomal dominant pattern of inheritance has been reported in a family harboring a C9ORF72 pathogenic mutation.

In summary, not all patients referred for memory complaints actually present an amnesic syndrome. Attentive clinicians should consider PPA and particularly svPPA in their differential when patients present progressive word-finding difficulties in their spontaneous speech. In addition to the fact that existing symptomatic drugs for AD are inefficient in svPPA and should be avoided, these patients could benefit from early speech-language pathologist interventions, such as language training, adoption of alternative communication strategies, and family support. Moreover, interventional research protocols with repetitive transcranial magnetic stimulation are ongoing in specialized centers to stimulate brain language regions in neurodegenerative aphasia. Finally, early identification of svPPA patients is critical for possible referral in future clinical trials testing molecules against TDP43 proteinopathies.

References

1. Gorno-Tempini ML, Hillis AE, Weintraub S, et al. Classification of primary progressive aphasia and its variants. *Neurology*. 2011;76 (11):1006–1014.

2. Patterson K, Nestor PJ, Rogers TT. Where do you know what you know? The representation of semantic knowledge in the human brain. *Nat Rev Neurosci*. 2007;8 (12):976–987.

3. Brambati SM, Amici S, Racine CA, et al. Longitudinal gray matter contraction in three variants of primary progressive aphasia: a tenser-based morphometry study. *Neuroimage Clin*. 2015;8:345–355.

4. Vitali P, Rouleau I, Deschaintre Y, et al. Proper name anomia in post-stroke aphasics: evidence from a multiple-case study. *Neurocase*. 2015;21(5): 563–572.

5. Bozzo F, Mirra A, Carrì MT. Oxidative stress and mitochondrial damage in the pathogenesis of ALS: new perspectives. *Neurosci Lett*. 2017;636: 3–8.

Obsessive Mandala Drawing in Semantic Dementia

Eline Donders and Yolande Pijnenburg

19.1 Main Complaint

A 65-year-old retired nurse with problems in following and remembering conversation.

19.2 Clinical History

Our patient is a retired nurse who visited the memory clinic of the VUmc Alzheimer Center at the age of 65. Her general practitioner referred her because of progressive forgetfulness over the past 5 years. Her medical history was unremarkable and except for some over-the-counter vitamin capsules, she did not use any medication. Other than memory complaints she also expressed having difficulty understanding what others were saying and the inability to recognize familiar faces. Moreover, her family reported loss of empathy and initiative and compulsive-like behaviors in her daily life. She had become compulsively engaged in cycling a fixed route during 1 hour every day and watched the same television programs every evening. Notably she played more music than she used to, although she did not seem to know the meaning of written musical notes. She used to visit museums for a hobby, but she now liked to draw mandalas in her free time. Since this took her several hours per day, she stayed up until late at night while drawing mandalas.

19.3 Examination

Neurological examination was normal, she was right-handed, and there were no eye movement disorders or extrapyramidal symptoms. She was euphoric and slightly disinhibited. Her Mini-Mental State Examination (MMSE) score was 28/30. There was a strong loss of semantic knowledge of both a verbal and nonverbal nature. In addition, there was mild executive dysfunction.

19.4 Diagnostic Workup

The MRI of the brain (Figure 19.1) revealed asymmetric left anterior temporal lobe atrophy, involving the parahippocampal gyrus with more prominent left than right hippocampal atrophy (Scheltens scale 2 versus 1).

19.5 Follow-Up

During clinical follow-up every 6 months, she developed a clear semantic language disorder, more emotional disinhibition, and rituals in the daily pattern. At night she spent several hours drawing mandalas (Figure 19.2), producing over 100 mandalas each month. Over time, these pictures became less complex and after being able to design them by heart, she became only able to copy them, but still with a perfect visuospatial structure. Several years later, however, she failed to draw her own mandalas, but she remained coloring them frequently. About 8 years after diagnosis a symptomatic treatment with trazodone 100 mg 2bd was started for disturbing and incontrollable behaviors such as strong agitation, shouting, screaming, and counting out loud. Initially this medication had beneficial effect, but after a few months it had to be replaced by olanzapine. Eventually she was placed in a nursing home and passed away in tranquility.

19.6 Discussion

Occurrence of visual and musical creativity in the setting of neurologic diseases has been reported in patients with semantic variant primary progressive aphasia, also called semantic dementia. Semantic dementia is a clinical subtype of frontotemporal dementia with asymmetrical degeneration of language-dominant anterior temporal lobe structures.

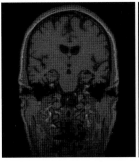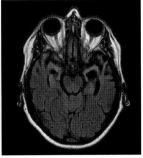

Figure 19.1 Coronal and transverse MRI images. Aymmetric left anterior temporal lobe atrophy, involving the parahippocampal gyrus with more prominent left than right hippocampal atrophy (Scheltens scale 2 versus 1).

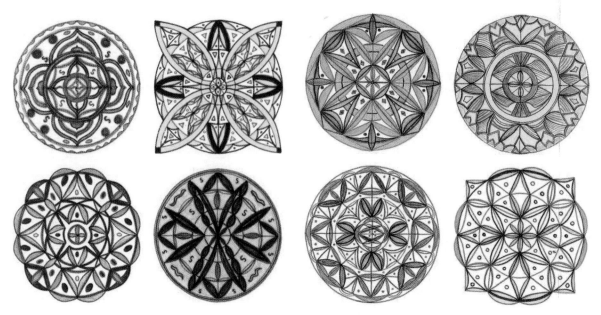

Figure 19.2 Examples of mandala drawings.

It is a language disorder that involves changes in the ability to speak, write, read, and understand what others are saying. Patients demonstrate a progressive deterioration of understanding words and recognizing objects while other cognitive functions remain remarkably spared. Their fluent empty speech becomes increasingly difficult to understand while they are not able to generate the key words in sentences. Unlike other FTD subtypes, semantic PPA generally does not produce changes in behavior or personality until later stages of the disease. Most people with progressive aphasia maintain the ability to care for themselves, keep up outside interests, and, sometimes, even remain employed for a few years after onset of the disorder. The average disease duration, from the onset of the illness is 8–10 years. Behavioral changes, including mental rigidity and loss of empathy occur in later stages. It is hypothesized that slow degeneration of language-dominant anterior temporal lobe brain function, provides remodeling of the nondominant hemisphere posterior structures.[1] The left parietal and left temporal lobe have inhibitory effects on free artistic expression through attention to respectively visuospatial detail and semantic labeling. Frontal executive functions are required for artistic expression, particularly right dorsolateral frontal initiation of a network for experimental behavior.

Activation of right posterior hemisphere structures could generate "de novo" artistic creativity.[2] Compulsive features in subtypes of frontotemporal dementia can also contribute to emergent creativity. In general, a rigid focus, perseverance, and precision are features of artistic creativity. Compulsive-like behaviors can manifest as repetitive artistic behavior as occurred in our patient. The "de novo" artistic creativity presented in our patient is hypothesized to be due to activation of right posterior hemisphere structures. While there is clear asymmetrical atrophy in the language-dominant left anterior temporal lobe. She also shows to have frontal compulsive behavior not only in her daily routine but most of all in her art work. The repetitive character of the art represents a need to organize thoughts and actions. The use of intense colors with perseverative and repetitive copying of similar patterns is an expression of being less constrained by learned rules as is seen in patients with frontal behavioral symptoms. There are several published clinical cases reporting a change in the artistic abilities in patients with neurological diseases, but no specific mention of drawing mandalas. A common notion suggests that losing control, especially relaxing social and emotional inhibitions or conventions, may favor personal expression and creativity. This case report underlines the hypothesis that disproportionate functional prevalence of the right over the left temporal lobe contributes to emergent creativity. Since communication abilities decrease in later stages of semantic dementia, this connection of neurological changes with art expression can be useful in accompanying SD patients in daily life.

References

1. Seeley WW, Matthews BR, Crawford RK, et al. Unraveling Bolero: progressive aphasia, transmodal creativity and the right posterior neocortex. *Brain.* 2008;131:39–49.

2. Miller BL, Boone K, Cummings JL, Read SL, Mishkin F. Functional correlates of musical and visual ability in frontotemporal dementia. *Br J Psychiatry.* 2000;176:458–463.

Forced into Retirement

Antoine Duquette, Philippe Huot, and Michel Panisset

20.1 Clinical History – Main Complaint

A 70-year-old man was referred because his balance had deteriorated in recent months. While he had only occasionally fallen over the previous 3 years, he now described a strong and consistent tendency to fall backward. He planned to retire as soon as possible partly because of this issue, but also because his productivity at work had decreased. His wife noted that he had been uncharacteristically impatient at home, but denied any memory difficulties.

20.2 General History

At the time of the initial evaluation, the patient was still employed and worked for a charity. He lived with his wife. He had never smoked or used recreational drugs. He drank one to two glasses of wine per day, three to four times a week. He had been diagnosed with hypertension and dyslipidemia for which he was treated with angiotensin conversion enzyme (ACE) and HMG-CoA reductase inhibitors, respectively. He had no urinary symptoms and denied erectile dysfunction.

20.3 Family History

The patient's father passed away at the age of 63 from a myocardial infarction. His mother died at the age of 88 with a diagnosis of Alzheimer's disease. She was also known for hypertension and dyslipidemia.

The patient had one sister who was 66 years old and in good health. He had one brother who suffered from bipolar disorder and committed suicide at the age of 35. He had one child, a 40-year-old son, who was in good health.

20.4 General Examination

The patient offered good cooperation but was somewhat apathetic. General examination including vital signs was normal. There was no orthostatic hypotension.

Neurological examination was characterized by poverty of movement and speech. There was striking hypomimia with a significant reduction in blinking. There was mild symmetrical lid retraction. Horizontal saccadic intrusions were observed upon visual fixation. Ocular smooth pursuit was complete, but horizontal pursuit was mildly saccadic and vertical pursuit was slow. Vertical pursuit was improved by the vestibular ocular reflex (VOR). There was no nystagmus. Voluntary vertical ocular saccades were impossible to obtain. Rigidity was prominent in the neck, while it was only seen with reinforcement in the limbs. There was no tremor at rest or during action. Strength was normal. Reflexes were normal and symmetrical. Sensory and cerebellar examinations were also normal. Gait was not wide-based, but the patient was very unstable upon turning and there was no postural response on the pull-test.

Montreal Cognitive Assessment (MoCA) score was 26/30. Executive function was affected as evidenced by multiple errors in Trail Making Test-B and reduced verbal fluency. The patient also had a tendency to persevere on the go-no-go test and was unable to copy a cube. Memory and orientation were not affected. There was no aphasia nor apraxia. When asked to clap his hands three times, the patient clapped six times.

20.5 Special Studies

Routine biochemical and hematological tests were normal.

Magnetic resonance imaging (MRI) of the brain showed mild leukoencephalopathy, proportional to what is observed in the patient's age group. A [18F]-fluoro-deoxyglucose (FDG) positron emission tomography (PET) revealed global cerebral hypometabolism with a relative predominance in the frontal lobes.

20.6 Diagnosis

The initial diagnosis was based upon clinical presentation. The combination of postural instability, apathy, marked axial rigidity, and severe abnormalities of vertical ocular saccades strongly suggested progressive supranuclear palsy (PSP). The axial rigidity was not in favor of late-onset Niemann-Pick type C disease. Central nervous system Whipple disease was considered unlikely because the patient did not have systemic symptoms such as arthralgia or weight loss. The absence of autonomic or cerebellar dysfunction along with early cognitive problems did not support a diagnosis of multiple system atrophy (MSA). The lack of asymmetry and apraxia was not suggestive of corticobasal degeneration (CBD). Dementia with Lewy bodies (DLB) was also unlikely given the absence of fluctuations and visual hallucinations.

20.7 Follow-Up

The patient did not respond to 600 mg of levodopa per day. Side effects prevented us from increasing the dosage further. We were thus unable to push the drug trial to 1,500 mg/day. Over the next 2 years, his balance deteriorated quickly and he became wheelchair-bound. Over the following 3 years, speech became unintelligible and he became dependent for most activities of daily living. By then, dysphagia was a significant problem and he was admitted twice for aspiration pneumonia. A dietician and a speech therapist suggested a percutaneous gastrostomy to reduce the risk of aspiration, but this was declined by the family. A year later, he succumbed to another episode of pneumonia. On histology, the substantia nigra showed significant neuronal loss, as well as gliosis. Tau-positive inclusions were observed in neurons (globose neurofibrillary tangles), astrocytes (tufted astrocytes), and oligodendrocytes (coiled bodies). The neuropathologist confirmed the diagnosis of PSP.

20.8 Discussion

PSP is an uncommon atypical parkinsonian syndrome first described in 1964 by Steele, Richardson, and Olczewski. Disease prevalence has been estimated between 5.8 and 6.5 per 100,000. While the diagnosis of definite PSP relies on histopathology, criteria for the clinical diagnosis of the disease include a gradually progressive disorder starting at the age of 40 or older, vertical supranuclear gaze palsy, and prominent postural instability with falls in the first year of onset.[1] Additional supportive features include axial akinesia or rigidity, abnormal neck posture often with marked retrocollis, poor response to levodopa, early dysphagia, and early dysarthria. Cognitive impairment typically occurs shortly after disease onset and is characterized by apathy, impairment of abstract thought, decreased verbal fluency, utilization or imitation behavior, and frontal release signs.[2]

However, in recent years, several PSP subgroups have been described in histologically confirmed PSP cases. In addition to classic PSP with Richardson's syndrome (PSP-RS), variants with predominant parkinsonism (PSP-P), pure akinesia with gait freezing (PSP-PAGF), corticobasal syndrome (PSP-CBS), progressive nonfluent aphasia (PSP-PNFA), predominant frontotemporal dysfunction (PSP-FTD), cerebellar ataxia (PSP-C), and primary lateral sclerosis (PSP-PLS) have been characterized (Table 20.1). While PSP-RS remains the most frequent syndrome, PSP-P may represent up to a third of PSP cases.

Early in the disease, it is often difficult to distinguish PSP from Parkinson's disease (PD), dementia with Lewy bodies (DLB), multiple system atrophy (MSA), and corticobasal degeneration (CBD). Magnetic resonance imaging (MRI) shows midbrain atrophy in 75–80% of PSP patients, but this feature is neither sensitive nor specific and tends to occur late in the disease. Several studies using a variety of structural measures have shown patterns that may prove helpful in the differential diagnosis of parkinsonian syndromes, but their clinical usefulness has yet to be confirmed.[5] Striatal dopamine transporter imaging (DaTscan) may be useful to distinguish PSP from controls and conditions which can mimic parkinsonism such as cerebrovascular disease and normal pressure hydrocephalus, but it is not superior to clinical evaluation to distinguish between parkinsonian syndromes. FDG-PET and tau imaging will probably be more useful in the future as diagnostic tools, but much work remains to be done to establish their sensitivity and specificity in the context of expanding PSP phenotypes. Highly specific cerebrospinal fluid (CSF) markers of PSP also are yet to emerge. In recent years, much progress has been made toward a better understanding of the genetics underlying PSP. While most cases are still considered sporadic, mutations in *MAPT*, which encodes for the tau protein and *LRRK2* have been uncovered in familial cases. Furthermore, a PSP-like presentation has been associated with mitochondrial diseases as well as mutations in *PRGN*, *C9orf72*, *CHMP2B*, *FUS*, *DCTN1*, *ATP13A2*, *NPC1*, *GBA*, and *PRNP*.

Table 20.1 Clinical features of PSP variants

	PSP-RS	PSP-P	PSP-PAGF	PSP-CBS	PSP-PNFA	PSP-FTD	PSP-C	PSP-PLS [4]
Rigidity	Axial > limb	Limb > axial	Axial	Limb > axial	+	+	Axial > limb	Limb > axial
Early postural instability and/or falls	+++	−	+	−/+	−	−	+++	+
Early eye movement abnormalities	+++	++	−/+	++	+	+	+++	+
Early cognitive decline	++	−	−	+++	+++	+++	++	+
Early frontal behavior	++	−	−	++	++	+++	++	+
Nonfluent aphasia and/or apraxia of speech	+	−	−	++	+++	++	−	−/+
Limb dystonia	+	+	−/+	+++	+	+	−	+
Pyramidal signs	+	+	+	++	+	+	−	+++
Levodopa response	−	++	−	−	−	−	−	−
Dysautonomia	−	−	−	−	−	−	−	−/+

Source: Adapted from [3].
−: absent, −/+: rare, +: occasional or mild, ++: usual or moderate, +++: frequent or severe.

20.9 Take-Home Messages

Executive dysfunction associated with axial parkinsonism and falls early in the disease should raise the possibility of progressive supranuclear palsy (PSP).

The complete neurological examination of a patient presenting with dementia should include vertical ocular saccades. This simple test may unmask PSP, but it can also direct clinicians toward treatable causes of cognitive impairment such as Whipple's disease and Niemann-Pick type C.

The range of clinical and cognitive PSP phenotypes is expanding. Apathy, impulsivity, and executive dysfunction have been classically described in PSP-RS. However, presentations with prominent cognitive features including corticobasal syndrome (CBS), progressive nonfluent aphasia (PNFA), and the behavioral variant of frontotemporal degeneration (FTD) have recently been associated with PSP histology.

Financial Disclosure

Dr. Duquette has received speaker fee and travel reimbursements from Actelion Pharmaceutiques Canada.

References

1. Litvan I, Agid Y, Calne D, et al. Clinical research criteria for the diagnosis of progressive supranuclear palsy (Steele-Richardson-Olszewski syndrome): report of the NINDS-SPSP international workshop. *Neurology*. 1996;47: 1–9.

2. Burrell JR, Hodges JR, Rowe JB. Cognition in corticobasal syndrome and progressive supranuclear palsy: a review. *Mov Disord*. 2014;29: 684–693.

3. Ling H. Clinical approach to progressive supranuclear palsy. *J Mov Disord.* 2016;9: 3–13.

4. Respondek G, Höglinger GU. The phenotypic spectrum of progressive supranuclear palsy. *Parkinsonism Relat Disord.* 2016;22: S34–S36.

5. Liscic RM, Srulijes K, Gröger A, Maetzler W, Berg D. Differentiation of progressive supranuclear palsy: clinical, imaging and laboratory tools. *Acta Neurol Scand.* 2013;127:362–370.

Who Are These People in My Living Room?

Fábio Henrique de Gobbi Porto and Ricardo Nitrini

21.1 Case Report

A 73-year-old right-handed man presented with a 1-year history of visual hallucinations. The hallucinations were described as the sight of intruders, about 20–30 people who were seen in his living-room and sometimes threaten him with their eyes. He frequently asked his wife about these people and how she could tolerate their presence. He also made complaints to the front door clerks about allowing these people to enter the building. Sometimes he saw children and animals running around the house. The hallucinations were vivid, well-formed and exclusively visual. He often had psychomotor agitation in response to the visions. Associated with the hallucinations, he began to present forgetfulness described as difficulties in word finding, decreased speed of thought, difficulty reasoning, occasional difficulties in understanding long sentences, and difficulty in learning new information. His relatives noted difficulties in recognition of objects through vision and intense fluctuation in the level of attention, with periods when the patient "stared at the walls" and periods of daytime drowsiness. He had an episode of topographical disorientation where he could not find his way back home. His clinical picture was described as slowly progressive.

The patient was evaluated in another service for the hallucinations, being prescribed a selective serotonin reuptake inhibitor (paroxetine), with worsening of the symptoms. After that, he received low doses of a typical neuroleptic (haloperidol – dose 0.5 mg/day), but had early impregnation symptoms (severe stiffness and bradykinesia) and had to discontinue the medication. During a hospitalization to investigate acute worsening of cognition, he received promethazine and risperidone through psychomotor agitation. Again, he had severe stiffness and drowsiness.

Neurologic examination showed bradykinesia in repetitive movements of the fingers in the left hand with mild stiffness and cogwheel rigidity, which could be caused by previous use of antipsychotics. He also had ideomotor apraxia for transitive (object-related) pantomime gestures. On cognitive evaluation, he scored 18/30 in the Mini-Mental State Examination (MMSE) (time orientation: 2/5; spatial orientation: 4/5;

immediate memory: 1/3; attention and calculation: 1/5; evocation: 2/3; naming 2/2; repetition of sentence: 1/1; verbal command: 3/3; written command: 1/1; phrase: 1/1; copy of the pentagons: 0/1). He also had impaired late recall on visual memory, reduced semantic fluency (animals), and visuospatial/executive impairments on the clock-drawing test (Figure 21.1). His score in the Functional Activities Questionnaire (FAQ) was 18. In this questionnaire, score ranges from 0 to 30, with higher scores being indicative of functional impairment.[1]

Magnetic resonance imaging depicted diffuse mild atrophy, more intense in medial temporal lobes (more evident to the right side) and mild, non-confluent white matter hyperintensities. Fluorodeoxyglucose positron emission tomography (FDG-PET) demonstrated bilateral asymmetrical (right more than left) hypometabolism in the temporal and parietal lobes with posterior extension to the occipital lobes (Figure 21.2).

21.2 Diagnosis

The main findings in this case were cognitive impairment with well-formed visual hallucinations and evident fluctuations of attention and alertness. Besides, early changes in visuospatial function (difficulty in the copy of the pentagons of the MMSE and very poor performance in the clock design) and extreme sensitivity to neuroleptic medications (early impregnation with low doses of haloperidol and possible neuroleptic syndrome with promethazine and risperidone) had been observed. Even in the absence of spontaneous (nondrug induced) parkinsonism, these features must be a red flag to the diagnosis of Lewy body dementia (LBD).[2–5] LBD is considered the second most frequent cause of degenerative dementia in the senile population (after Alzheimer's disease –

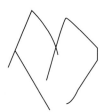

Figure 21.1 Copy of the pentagons (MMSE) and clock-drawing test in the first visit.

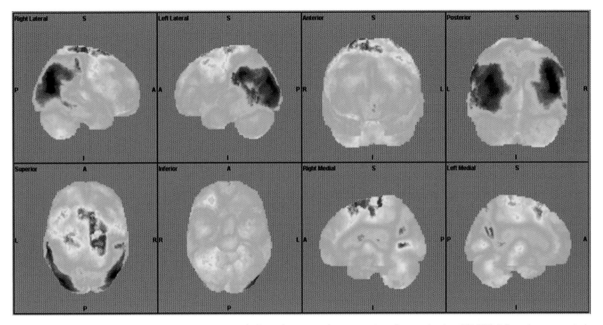

Figure 21.2 Fluorodeoxyglucose positron emission with three-dimensional stereotactic surface projection (3D-SSP): bilateral asymmetrical (right more than left) hypometabolism in the temporal and parietal lobes with posterior extension to the occipital lobes.

AD) and the third most frequent cause of dementia after AD and vascular dementia.[2–4] LBD is characterized by progressive cognitive decline in which memory may not be the main cognitive domain that is affected initially. Attention, executive functions, and visuospatial processing deficits are often the earliest impaired cognitive functions. In addition to cognitive impairment, central features include spontaneous parkinsonism, visual hallucinations, and fluctuation in arousal and alertness. Additionally, extreme sensitivity to neuroleptic medications, rapid eye movement (REM) sleep behavior disorder, daytime sleepiness, and dysautonomia can be found, in some cases, even before the cognitive and motor symptoms.[2,3,5]

LBD neuropathology is characterized by cortical and subcortical accumulation of Lewy bodies (LB), which are alpha-synuclein-positive intracytoplasmic neuronal inclusions, usually present in the monoaminergic and cholinergic nuclei of the brainstem in idiopathic Parkinson's disease (PD).[2–6] LBD is very similar to the dementia found in the advanced stages of PD, called Parkinson's Disease Dementia (PDD), but LBD usually manifests with more severe cognitive and neuropsychiatric impairment and less severe motor symptoms. The "one year" rule has been used

to differentiate the two entities, but in clinical practice this didactical split is difficult to apply.[5] If the cognitive symptoms precede or appear in the first year of the motor symptoms, it is classified as LBD. In cases where the cognitive deficit begins after the first year of motor symptoms, the diagnosis is PDD. This division is arbitrary and probably both entities represent the spectrum of a clinical-pathological continuum.

LBD is characterized by an intense and precocious cholinergic deficit, and some of the symptoms may be more clearly responsive to anticholinesterase medications, at least in the initial clinical phases when compared with AD.[7]

21.3 Treatment and Follow-Up

After establishing the diagnosis of LBD, the acetylcholinesterase inhibitor rivastigmine was introduced orally with progressive increases in total dosage. After gradual increase of rivastigmine, reaching 12 mg/day, the patient presented gradual reduction of visual hallucinations and fluctuations of arousal and attention. He began to exhibit insight into hallucinations, realizing most of the time that they were not real and was no longer agitated by them. Two months after the introduction of rivastigmine, relatives reported a substantial cognitive improvement. The MMSE score increased to 25. Six months after starting the treatment, family reported that hallucinations became rare, episodes of fluctuation in wakefulness disappeared, and there was improvement in the ability to do daily tasks. At this visit, the scores were 26 in the MMSE and 14 in the FAQ. His visuospatial and visuoconstructive abilities may have had a small improvement, but were still very impaired (Figure 21.3).

About 1 year after starting treatment, the patient began to present gait difficulties, imbalance, and the hallucinations returned, causing agitation again. On this occasion, the neurological examination showed gait with anterior flexion of the trunk and reduction of the associated movements of the arms, postural instability with retropulsion in the "pull test", increased hypertonia, and bradykinesia in the hands. In addition, he presented worsening of the ideomotor apraxia and appearance of apraxia of imitation. The MMSE score was 24. Even though he was using rivastigmine 12 mg/day (maximum recommended oral dose), the dosage was increased to 15 mg/day (he could not tolerate the transdermical preparation due to an allergic skin reaction). There was again a decrease in visual hallucinations and cognitive benefits. The patient tolerated well the increased dosage, without cholinergic side effects. Memantine 20 mg/day was also introduced. After 2 years of follow-up, the MMSE score was 22, hallucinations and fluctuations in wakefulness remained under control when he suffered a severe car accident, which caused traumatism to the cervical spine. He was submitted to tracheostomy and remained in the intensive care unit for 2 weeks and in the hospital for 2 months. Since then he was treated at his hometown where he gradually recovered from the traumatisms and had a transitory period of moderate control of the hallucinations with rivastigmine 18 mg/day, olanzapine 1.25 mg/day, and low doses of levodopa. He died

with severe dementia 6 years after the beginning of the symptoms of the LBD.

21.4 Discussion

This case exemplifies that types of dementia, especially LBD, present a favorable response to anticholinesterase medication, at least initially. This response is manifest both in cognitive and neuropsychiatric symptoms. Functional improvement is sometimes clearly observed.

Cholinergic deficiency is a hallmark of several dementias including AD and LBD.[7,8] Studies with toxins that selectively injure the nucleus basalis of Meynert, the main cholinergic projection nucleus to the cortex, demonstrated deficits in memory and attention (sustained and divided attention). The loss of cholinergic neurons and decreased levels of choline acetyltransferase is much more severe and precocious in LBD when compared with AD. In addition, medications with anticholinergic properties may cause hallucinations and altered arousal and alertness, symptoms often found in LBD. Not surprisingly, acetylcholinesterase inhibitors improve hallucinations, wakefulness fluctuations, and attention in patients with LBD, often more intensely than in other dementias. Cholinergic deficiency is a critical factor for the manifestations of symptoms in the early stage of LBD, explaining the greater response to anticholinesterases, but may be less important in the early stages of AD.[2,4] This highlights the importance of the differential diagnosis in the early stages of the dementia syndromes, because with the progression of AD and consequent greater cholinergic deficit, similar symptoms of LBD can occur, making differential diagnosis difficult in late stages. Regarding the clinical progression of the disease, studies have shown a faster rate of decline of LBD in relation to AD, with the extrapyramidal symptoms being strong predictors of morbidity and mortality.[2–4]

Oftentimes, differential diagnosis in early stages of LBD is challenging. Clinical symptoms may be subtle and similar to other diseases. Visuospatial impairment and visual hallucinations are considered an early clinical tip to suspect LBD.[9,10] Also, posterior parietal and occipital hypometabolism in FDG-PET is suggestive of LBD,[10] sometimes remembering the metabolic pattern found in posterior cortical atrophy syndrome,[11,12] as we saw in this

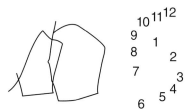

Figure 21.3 Copy of the pentagons (MMSE) and clock-drawing test on follow up.

case (Figure 21.2). Biomarkers in the cerebrospinal fluid (CSF) usually do not help distinguish between LBD and AD because low levels of β-amyloid, and high levels of tau and phosphorylated-tau may be found in both diseases, but may help in differentiation of LBD from PDD.[13,14] Preliminary data have shown decreased levels of CSF alpha-synuclein in synucleinopathies in comparison with AD, but the specificity was low, in spite of good positive predictive value.[15] Specific alpha-synuclein measurements still need to be validated to clinical practice.[15] However, specific CSF biomarkers are greatly needed for better outcomes in disease-modifying treatments approaches.[16]

Sometimes, additional benefit can be seen with supramaximal dosages of acetylcholinesterase inhibitors, as we demonstrated in our patient. In certain dementias, due to intense cholinergic deficit, this strategy may be effective and well tolerated. Clinical benefits may clearly outweigh the risks of side effects. Additional treatments with atypical antipsychotics targeting psychotic symptoms and dopaminergic replacement are often necessary. Due to the possibility of worsening extrapyramidal symptoms and

hallucinations, these medications must be prescribed with caution. In this case, dopaminergic replacement therapy was considered about 1 year after treatment when parkinsonian signs became more severe. However, severe hallucinations causing agitation had returned and we thought it would be better to increase the doses of acetylcholinesterase inhibitor than to start levodopa, which may cause and increase hallucinations. It should be stressed that most of the time, it is possible to use simultaneously acetylcholinesterase inhibitor and levodopa, when one starts with low doses of levodopa.

21.5 Take-Home Message

LBD is a relatively frequent form of dementia, which presents cognitive impairment, parkinsonism, and neuropsychiatric symptoms. LBD is characterized by an intense and precocious cholinergic deficit, even in the initial stages, providing a target for anticholinesterase medication therapy. Sometimes there is benefit with supramaximal doses, with good tolerance. Correct diagnosis is important for therapeutic planning and follow-up of cases.

References

1. Pfeffer RI, Kurosaki TT, Harrah CH Jr, Chance JM, Filos S. Measurement of functional activities in older adults in the community. *J Gerontol.* 1982;37:323–329.

2. McKeith IG, Dickson DW, Lowe J, et al. Diagnosis and management of dementia with Lewy bodies: third report of the DLB consortium. *Neurology.* 2005;65:1863–1872.

3. Ferman TJ, Boeve BF. Dementia with Lewy bodies. *Neurol Clin.* 2007;25:741–760.

4. Brucki SMD, Magaldi RM, Morillo LS, et al. *Demências: Enfoque multidisciplinary das bases fisiopatológicas ao diagnóstico e tratamento.* São Paulo: Editora Atheneu; 2011.

5. Mega MS, Masterman DL, Benson DF, et al. Dementia with Lewy bodies: reliability and validity of clinical and pathologic criteria. *Neurology.* 1996;47:1403–1409.

6. Torres EM, Perry TA, Blockland A, et al. Behavioural, histochemical and biochemical consequences of selective immunolesions in discrete regions of the basal forebrain cholinergic system. *Neuroscience.* 1994;63:95–122.

7. Tiraboschi P, Hansen LA, Alford M, et al. Early and widespread cholinergic losses differentiate dementia with Lewy bodies from Alzheimer disease. *Arch Gen Psychiatry.* 2002;59:946–951.

8. McKeith I, Mintzer J, Aarsland D, et al, on behalf of the International Psychogeriatric Association Expert Meeting on DLB. Dementia with Lewy bodies. *Lancet Neurol.* 2004;3:19–28.

9. Li X, Rastogi P, Gibbons JA, Chaudhury S. Visuo-cognitive skill deficits in Alzheimer's disease and Lewy body disease: a comparative analysis. *Ann Indian Acad Neurol.* 2014;17:12–18.

10. Tiraboschi P, Salmon DP, Hansen LA, et al. What best differentiates Lewy body from Alzheimer's disease in early-stage dementia? *Brain.* 2006;129:729–735.

11. Ishii K. PET approaches for diagnosis of dementia. *AJNR Am J Neuroradiol.* 2014;35:2030–2038.

12. Beh SC, Muthusamy B, Calabresi P, et al. Hiding in plain sight: a closer look at posterior cortical atrophy. *Pract Neurol.* 2015;15:5–13.

13. Andersson M, Zetterberg H, Minthon L, Blennow K, Londos E. The cognitive profile and CSF biomarkers in dementia with Lewy bodies and Parkinson's disease dementia. *Int J Geriatr Psychiatry.* 2011;26:100–105.

14. Schade S, Mollenhauer B. Biomarkers in biological fluids for

dementia with Lewy bodies. *Alzheimers Res Ther.* 2014; 6:72.

15. Mollenhauer B, Locascio JJ, Schulz-Schaeffer W, et al. α-Synuclein and tau concentrations in cerebrospinal fluid of patients presenting with parkinsonism: a cohort study. *Lancet Neurol.* 2011;10:230–240.

16. Kim D, Kim YS, Shin DW, Park CS, Kang JH. Harnessing cerebrospinal fluid biomarkers in clinical trials for treating Alzheimer's and Parkinson's diseases: potential and challenges. *J Clin Neurol.* 2016;12:381–392.

Case of Parkinsonism That Never Had a Good Response to Levodopa

Frédéric Potvin Gingras, Antoine Duquette, Philippe Huot,
and Michel Panisset

22.1 Clinical History – Main Complaint

This 62-year-old former accountant presented to a neurologist with complaints of a right hand tremor, slowness, and gait difficulties. He was diagnosed with Parkinson's disease (PD) and received pramipexole up to 1.5 mg tid. On this medication, he reported being well for 2 years. After 3 years of evolution, levodopa/carbidopa was introduced because of a worsening of his parkinsonism. His tremor was initially significantly improved by levodopa, but the effect was lost after less than a year. Higher doses caused episodes of hypotension and also spasms of his neck and toes which were treated with clonazepam. At the fifth year, he developed significant freezing of gait and needed a walker to ambulate safely.

The patient never seemed to have motor fluctuations or end-of-dose wearing off. In addition, he complained of a muffled voice, dry mouth, nycturia at least three times per night, incontinence at times, and dream enactment. He admitted having erectile dysfunction for some years before his diagnosis. Recently, he was reported not to participate in social gatherings as he had before, and he seemed not to have interest in any activities be it at home or outside. He had been diagnosed with a depressive disorder for which he was taking citalopram. All his symptoms lead to a gradual loss of autonomy. He was eventually sent to a movement disorder clinic for medication optimization.

Upon further questioning both him and his wife, it was found that he had left to his wife most of his household responsibilities including the finances, a significant factor for an accountant. Although it was not initially clear whether this was due to his apathy or to cognitive deficits, it became clear that he had significant cognitive impairments including not being able to be trusted to take his medications and to keep track of his appointments. His wife described a generalized disorganization. He had to retire earlier than he wished because he felt he did not have the energy to follow the accounts of his clientele.

22.2 General History

The patient was married and the couple had two healthy children. His past medical history was remarkable for a von Willebrand disease and two discal hernias. Years ago, he also had a cholecystectomy. His medication consisted of tamsulosin, clonazepam, citalopram, sildenafil, baclofen, pramipexole (1.5 mg TID), and levodopa/carbidopa 100/25 six times per day.

22.3 Family History

Both his parents died of heart disease in their early seventh decade. The patient had an older brother who had had a coronary artery bypass at age 57 and an older sister who died of breast cancer at age 66. There was no history of PD or other neurological disease in the family.

22.4 Examination

Vital signs were notable for orthostatic hypotension with a drop of systolic blood pressure of more than 30 mmHg without tachycardia on multiple measuring. Blood pressure was otherwise at 105/70. Heart rate was unremarkable. Cardiopulmonary exam was normal.

The patient was alert and cooperating well. Bedside cognitive testing revealed a mild disorientation in time, general slowing of thought processes, diminished verbal fluency, recall difficulties that were improved by cues, and distractibility. He also had impairments on figure drawing and copying. His score on the Montreal Cognitive Assessment (MoCA) was 21/30, and the test was fairly long to pass. On the clock drawing, the numbers were spaced unevenly and included supplementary numbers.

Cranial nerve examination revealed slow, jerky ocular pursuit but no gaze limitations or saccade anomalies. The patient had hypomimia, dysphagia while attempting to drink out of a glass of water, and a dysphonia with a peculiar quivering voice and an increased pitch.

Parkinsonism was present, heralded by symmetrical mild to moderate rigidity and bradykinesia of the upper and lower limbs. A slightly asymmetrical jerky postural and action tremor of the upper limbs was noted. It nearly disappeared at rest. Gait was notable for a stooped posture, slowness, occasional freezing, decomposed half-turn, and diminished arm swing. Although the patient did not fall, he was unstable without his cane and showed retropulsion. Examiners were not able to note any motor fluctuations throughout the interview even though the patient was near the time of his next levodopa dose.

Strength was normal. There were no sensory impairments or ataxia. The stretch muscle reflexes were increased at 3/4 all over and the plantar responses showed Babinski signs.

22.5 Laboratory Studies

Routine blood tests were normal. Olfaction testing with the "Sniffin' Sticks" odor identification test (SS-12) was at normal level for age. Magnetic resonance imaging (MRI) of the brain showed T2 hypointensity of the posterior aspect of the putamen with a hyperintense lateral rim.

He was sent for a neuropsychological evaluation which revealed changes compatible with a major neurocognitive disorder characterized mainly by executive and visuospatial dysfunctions. Deficits were noted in attention with sensitivity to interference, in task initiation and planning, in working memory, in mental flexibility during graphic series or trail making test, and in visuospatial functions with the Rey figure and the parallel lines. Memory was less impaired, as was semantic knowledge, although encoding and chronologic sequence of memories were affected.

22.6 Diagnosis

The clinical picture of parkinsonism, depression, and rapid eye movement behavior disorder (RBD) was suggestive of a synucleinopathy. His unsustained response to levodopa, the early and prominent autonomic dysfunction and the early postural instability suggested a diagnosis of multiple system atrophy with predominant parkinsonism subtype (MSA-P). The imaging abnormalities were other features that would support this impression. The absence of gaze limitations made the alternate diagnosis of progressive supranuclear palsy (PSP) less likely, as did the absence of apraxia and the presence of RBD for a diagnosis of

corticobasal degeneration. The transient response to levodopa and the jerky postural tremor made a diagnosis of PD also unlikely.

22.7 Evolution

Levodopa was increased to the maximum tolerated dose and dopamine agonists were progressively withdrawn. Orthostatic hypotension was addressed with domperidone and midodrine. The alpha-blocker tamsulosin was ceased for the risk of worsening hypotension and was replaced by solifenacin. His urinary problems were initially treated with mirabegron but later needed intravesical injections of botulinum toxin. Patient was referred to physiotherapy and occupational therapy for balance training and home adaptation.

Nevertheless, over the course of the next few years, he developed severe gait problems which forced him to a wheelchair and he was eventually bed bound. His instability was caused in part by camptocormia, retropulsion, and frequent uncontrollable syncope due to orthostatic hypotension. Axial and appendicular dystonia appeared. In addition to RBD, his sleep was further complicated by severe sleep apnea requiring CPAP. He slowly developed a peculiar respiratory bruit that became a high-pitched laryngeal stridor, worse during sleep. His dysphagia worsened to the point where he needed installation of a gastrojejunostomy to prevent aspiration.

He died at age 75 of respiratory complications, 13 years after the onset of his disease. Autopsy confirmed the diagnosis of MSA-P.

22.8 Discussion

This case was a typical example of MSA-P. MSA is a synucleinopathy of unknown etiology. No genetic factors have been confirmed to date, although an association has been described between MSA and mutations in the SNCA and COQ2 genes. The main clinical characteristics of the disease are akinetic parkinsonism, cerebellar signs, and dysautonomia.[1] MSA-P is the most frequent form of MSA in the Occident whereas MSA-C, the cerebellar form, is more frequent in Asia. MSA is a rare disease, with a prevalence of approximately 2–5/100,000, MSA-P subtype being two to four times more frequent. Median age at onset is 58 years old.

At first, MSA-P can be very difficult to differentiate from PD, more so than many other parkinsonian syndromes. The parkinsonism is often symmetrical and without tremors or with action tremors of higher frequency, sometimes with a jerky component. Postural instability commonly appears within 3 years of onset, but is less marked than in PSP. Hypophonia and monotonous speech is frequent but a distinct quivering voice with an increase in pitch is often noted. Response to levodopa therapy is present in only 20–50% of cases and is only transient. It can also greatly exacerbate dysautonomia and produce a characteristic unilateral orofacial dystonic spasm. Dysautonomia is present, not unlike in PD, but is often very early and out of proportion with the parkinsonism. Urogenital dysfunctions – incontinence, urgency or retention, and impotence for men – are often the presenting symptoms and are present in >80% of cases (nearly 100% for erectile dysfunction). Orthostatic hypotension is seen in >75% of patients and usually appears after urinary signs. Other common signs are prominent dysphagia, high-pitched stridor, pyramidal signs like Babinski's, other movement disorders like dystonia or myoclonus, anterocollis, Pisa syndrome, and RBD. People with MSA do not have olfactory deficits.[2]

Although cognitive functions are classically described as being spared in MSA, impairments resembling Parkinson's and PSP are increasingly recognized. As much as 20% of patients could be affected, even early in the disease, contrarily to what was once thought.[3] Executive, visuospatial, and constructional dysfunctions, deficits in attention, diminished verbal fluency and perseveration are the most common findings. Depression and anxiety disorders are frequent. Pseudobulbar affect has been described but is less common than in PSP.

Common findings on MRI imaging include atrophy of the putamen, pons and middle cerebellar peduncle as well as T2 hypointensity of the posterior putamen with hyperintensity of its lateral border depending on the subtype of MSA. T2 hyperintense signals can also be noted in the middle cerebellar peduncle and in the pons, where it can form a cross called the "hot cross bun sign." None of these findings are entirely specific and MRI can also be completely normal.[4] Positron emission tomography with FDG can show hypometabolism in the striatum, frontal lobe, brainstem, and cerebellum, but again this is probably not specific. DATscan will give results similar to PD and is thus of limited use. I-123 metaiodobenzylguanidine (MIBG) scintigraphy has demonstrated a reduced myocardial uptake in PD compared with MSA that could help distinguish them.[5] Other tests that might be useful include autonomic testing with the tilt-table or ambulatory blood pressure and heart rate monitoring, sweat testing with QSART, polysomnography, and urodynamic studies.

Definite diagnosis of MSA requires postmortem pathological confirmation. Macroscopic findings include olivo-ponto-cerebellar atrophy and loss of neurons, pallor of substantia nigra as well as atrophy and darkening of posterior putamen. Microscopic examination reveals inclusions of proteins including α-synuclein in the cytoplasm or nucleus of glial cells and neurons. Glial cytoplasmic inclusions are the hallmark of MSA and are required for diagnosis, and they correlate well with disease duration and severity.[2] Common sites where they accumulate include the putamen, substantia nigra, globus pallidus, pontine nuclei, locus ceruleus, reticular formation of the pons, and intermediolateral cell columns.

MSA progresses faster than PD, with an average life expectancy around 6–9 years from onset, but some patients can go well over 10 years.

22.9 Take-Home Message

MSA-P presents as an atypical form of PD with symmetrical parkinsonism, postural or action tremor, and early falls. Dysautonomic features, especially urogenital, are prominent and early. Response to dopamine replacement therapy is absent, partial, or short-lived. Whereas it was once thought that cognitive impairment was incompatible with the disease, it is now recognized that a subcortical frontal lobe dysfunction profile is not uncommon.

References

1. Gilman S, Wenning GK, Low PA, et al. Second consensus statement on the diagnosis of multiple system atrophy. *Neurology*. 2008;71(9): 670–676.

2. McFarland NR, Diagnostic approach to atypical parkinsonian syndromes. *Continuum*. 2016;22(4, Movement Disorders): 1117–1142.

3. Brown RG, Lacomblez L, Landwehrmeyer BG, et al.

Cognitive impairment in patients with multiple system atrophy and progressive supranuclear palsy. *Brain*. 2010;133(8):2382–2393.

4. Brooks DJ, Seppi K, Neuroimaging Working Group on MSA. Proposed neuroimaging criteria for the diagnosis of multiple system atrophy. *Mov Disord*. 2009;24(7): 949–964.

5. Treglia G, Stefanelli A, Cason E, et al. Diagnostic performance of iodine-123-metaiodobenzylguanidine scintigraphy in differential diagnosis between Parkinson's disease and multiple-system atrophy: a systematic review and a meta-analysis. *Clin Neurol Neurosurg*. 2011;113(10):823–829.

Common Complaints; Rare Pathology

Chris Feehan

23.1 Case Report

Mrs. A is a 30-year-old female who presented to the emergency department of a major urban hospital in Canada with complaints of abdominal pain, fatigue, and tremor. Her first language is Arabic and history taking was complicated by Mrs. A's very limited English. She had arrived in Canada only a few days before presentation. Before coming to Canada, Mrs. A lived for approximately 2 years in a refugee camp and had very limited access to medical care during that time.

Mrs. A was suffering from significant abdominal discomfort and distension and this was her primary complaint on presentation. The pain was diffuse but worse in the upper right quadrant. This pain was intermittent but had been worsening over the prior 6 months. She had also noticed worsening bilateral ankle swelling over a similar time period. There was associated fatigue and nausea but no jaundice or vomiting.

Once Arabic translation was obtained, it was revealed that she had an approximately 4-month history of tremors, stiffness, and reduced coordination in all four limbs. This was primarily in the arms and hands, although she also reported some unsteadiness in her gait. These symptoms were fluctuating but worsening steadily. Impairment was asymmetric, with the worst symptoms in the right arm. As a result of these symptoms, Mrs. A was having difficulty with household tasks including cooking and cleaning. She reported that she sometimes dropped things she was holding and felt she had reduced coordination. Mrs. A also reported weakness, especially in her right hand, although it was not clear whether this dysfunction was a result of her tremor or due to actual weakness. When her tremor was at its worst she was unable to feed herself. However, in between episodes of tremor her function was reasonably good and she experienced little to no functional impairment. The periods of worsening tremor and stiffness were becoming more frequent and at presentation were happening daily and lasting for hours at a time.

Mrs. A was also experiencing mild dysarthria for 1–2 months prior to presentation. There were no problems with swallowing. Finally, Mrs. A was also reporting pain in her extremities. The pain was described as aching and burning throughout her extremities but primarily in her right leg, focused on the right knee. Mrs. A had been experiencing this pain for many months with little progression. She was not taking any medication to treat the pain.

At this point, through translation and further review of her documents, it became clear that Mrs. A had been diagnosed with Wilson's disease since age 24. She had a sister who died at age 15 – apparently from complications of Wilson's disease. Prior to fleeing her home country and living in a refugee camp for 2 years, Mrs. A had been on zinc therapy. However, she had not had any access to medications during the years she lived in the refugee camp.

Mrs. A and her family denied any personality changes, behavior changes, mood disturbances, or hallucinations. She endorsed some difficulty with short-term memory and concentration over the last few months prior to presentation.

Physical exam demonstrated slightly dysarthric speech when speaking Arabic. Eye movements were unrestricted in any direction but smooth pursuit eye movements were saccadic. A sardonic smile was noted. When initially assessed by Ophthalmology, it was reported that Mrs. A did not have Kayser-Fleischer rings – visible deposits of copper in the Descemet's membrane of the eye – encircling the irises. This was the information available to the Neurology team at the time of assessment of the patient. However, this was likely due to limited examination tools and cooperation. Subsequent exam using a slit-lamp device revealed bilateral, dense Kayser-Fleischer rings. Examination of the remainder of cranial nerves was unremarkable.

Tone in the extremities was normal with no rigidity or cog-wheeling. Deep tendon reflexes were relatively brisk with some minor spreading. Strength was normal and symmetrical in all four limbs. There was a low amplitude and low-to-moderate frequency resting tremor in her right hand. Repetitive movements of the fingers and hands were unremarkable and her rate, rhythm, force, and amplitude were all normal. Gait was only mildly impaired, with some imbalance, especially during a tandem gait task. There was a decreased arm swing bilaterally, predominately on

Table 23.1 Selected lab results

Lab test	Value	Normal range
Ceruloplasmin	59 mg/L	200–500 mg/L
24-h Urinary Cu excretion	17.56 umol/day	<0.6 umol/day
Serum Cu	5.4 umol/L	11–26 -umol/L
Hemoglobin	105 g/L	123–157 g/L
Platelets	59 × 109/L	130–400 × 109/L
Alanine aminotransferase (ALT)	46 U/L	10–65 U/L
Aspartate aminotransferase (AST)	77 U/L	10–38 U/L
Alkaline phosphatase	128 U/L	30–135 U/L
Albumin	17 g/L	34–50 g/L

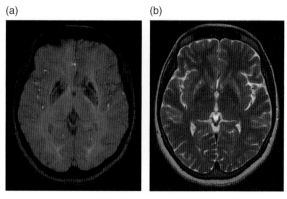

(a)   (b)

Figure 23.1 Brain MRI of a 30-year-old female with Wilson's disease. (a) MRI Susceptibility-weighted angiography (SWAN) sequence – demonstrates marked hypointensity of the bilateral basal ganglia, most pronounced in the putamina. (b) MRI T2 fast relaxation fast spin echo sequence (FRFSE) – demonstrates hyperintensity of the bilateral putamina corresponding with those areas seen as hypodense on SWAN sequence.

the right. She was able to walk without an assistive device. Sensory testing was unremarkable.

Mrs. A had mild abdominal distension with no detectable ascites. She was tender in the right upper quadrant. There was also moderate pitting pedal edema. Mrs. A had palmar erythema but no clubbing. No other stigmata of liver disease were appreciated.

Selected initial lab results are shown in Table 23.1. They revealed a low ceruloplasmin, high urinary Cu excretion and low serum Cu – suggestive of dysregulated Cu homeostasis. There was a mild normocytic anemia and significant thrombocytopenia. A liver panel demonstrated an elevated aspartate aminotransferase (AST) and low albumin – suggestive of liver dysfunction.

An abdominal ultrasound demonstrated liver cirrhosis, splenomegaly, and mild ascites. A non-contrast CT scan of the head showed subtle low attenuation changes in the basal ganglia bilaterally which were not specific or diagnostic. A follow-up MRI of the brain showed abnormalities in the basal ganglia with T1 and T2 hyperintensity and susceptibility-weighted angiography sequence (SWAN) hypointensity. These findings were particularly pronounced in the bilateral putamina. Representative slices of the patient's MRI are shown in Figure 23.1. These MRI findings were consistent with central nervous system (CNS) manifestations of Wilson's disease.

Given the relatively advanced nature of Mrs. A's disease and her years without treatment, chelating treatment for copper was initiated rapidly. The risk for neurological worsening with initiation of chelators was felt to be acceptable and was monitored. This phenomenon is discussed below. Trientene was not available for prescription in Canada, so treatment was initiated with D-penicillamine 500 mg orally three times daily. Pyridoxine (vitamin B6) supplementation was also initiated to prevent penicillamine-induced deficiency.

Mrs. A was also seen by the gastroenterology service for consideration of liver transplant. She was started on furosemide 40 mg twice daily and spironolactone 25 mg three times daily for diuresis of her ascites and pedal edema. Mrs. A continued to follow-up with the liver transplant team as an outpatient but at the time of publication had not been confirmed for the transplant list.

After a few months of treatment with high-dose penicillamine, Mrs. A was experiencing some improvement in her neurological symptoms. Her resting tremor of the right hand resolved, although she continued to have difficulties with coordination of the hands. Her sardonic smile also resolved. No significant neurological worsening was seen with her chelating treatment. If there is any future deterioration in her neurological symptoms zinc therapy was to be considered.

23.2 Discussion

Copper (Cu) is an element required in trace amounts in the human diet. This is primarily to act as a co-factor in the function of a number of essential proteins, enzymes, and metabolic processes.[1] These proteins have diverse functions including regulation of iron transport and utilization, synthesis and release of a number of essential proteins, and protection against free-radial damage to cells. As a result, copper homeostasis is a complex and tightly controlled process.

Ceruloplasmin is the primary transporter of Cu in the bloodstream.[1] The ATP7B protein catalyzes the incorporation of Cu into ceruloplasmin in the liver as well as assisting in the transport of Cu into bile for excretion. In Wilson's disease, a mutation in the gene for ATP7B leads to Cu accumulation and deposition in the liver. This results in free-radial damage and eventual fibrosis of the liver. Additionally, unbound Cu is released into the bloodstream where it deposits primarily in the brain, kidneys, and eyes.[2] In the brain, the deposits are primarily in the basal ganglia where they lead to more free-radial damage and eventual fibrosis.

Wilson's disease was first described by the British neurologist Dr. Samuel A. K. Wilson in 1912 as "progressive lenticular degeneration". It has an estimated prevalence of 1–3/30,000, with approximately 1/90 people carrying an abnormal ATP7B copy.[3] The disease is concentrated in some isolated populations but there is no significant regional or gender predilection.

Wilson's disease presents in one of three ways: neurologic, psychiatric, or hepatic. These presentations have a roughly equal incidence although psychiatric presentations of Wilson's are likely under-diagnosed.[3] There is a wide variety in presentation even between family members. The majority of cases present in young patients (5–35 years old). Older patients are more likely to present with neurologic manifestations.[2] The difference in presentation is suspected to be from a variety of factors including diet, different mutations, and variable penetrance.

Patients presenting with hepatic Wilson's disease have a range of disease at presentation. These range from asymptomatic to cirrhosis, portal hypertension, and/or acute hepatitis (often with hemolytic anemia).[4] Incidence of acute liver failure at presentation is estimated to be 5–17%.

There is also a diverse presentation of neurologic Wilson's disease.[2] The most common symptoms are dysarthria, ataxia, dystonia, tremor, and parkinsonism. Other less common symptoms reported include: risus sardonicus, chorea, athetosis, cognitive impairment, seizures, hyperreflexia, myoclonia, and dysautonomia.

A psychiatric presentation of Wilson's disease is most common in those patients who also have neurologic Wilson's, however psychiatric manifestations can be the only presenting symptoms and are likely under reported. Depression is the most common psychiatric presentation of Wilson's (20–30%). Other symptoms include: personality change, irritability, impulsiveness, labile mood, sexual disinhibition, inappropriate behavior, dysthymia, bipolar affective disorder, and psychosis.[4]

One well known manifestation of Wilson's is the presence of Kayser-Fleischer rings – visible deposits of copper in the Descemet's membrane of the eye – encircling the irises. Besides the brain, eyes, and liver, other organs which can be affected by Wilson's include: kidney, muscles, thyroid, pancreas, reproductive organs, and skin. This can cause symptoms such as fanconi syndrome, nephrolithiasis, arthropathy, gigantism, cardiomyopathy, myopathy, hypoparathyroidism, pancreatitis, impotence, infertility, blue lunulae, acanthosis nigricans, and pretibial hyperpigmentation.[5]

Due to its complex nature and diverse presentation, diagnosis of Wilson's disease starts with clinical suspicion and familiarity with the condition. The differential diagnosis is very broad and depends on the presenting symptoms. According to recent guidelines, Wilson's should be considered for any liver abnormality of unknown cause and should be specifically excluded for unexplained liver dysfunction along with a neurological or psychiatric disorder.[4] In general, younger age at presentation increases suspicion.

Initial tests to be performed include liver panel, CBC, serum ceruloplasmin, serum Cu, 24-hour urine Cu excretion, and an ocular slit-lamp exam. Further testing in cases of strong suspicion include a liver biopsy for quantitative Cu, genetic testing for ATP7B mutations, and a penicillamine challenge (looking for large increase in Cu excretion).

Clinicians should be aware of some significant limitations to serum ceruloplasmin testing.[4] Serum ceruloplasmin will be low in 85–90% of Wilson's patients but the test has a low positive predictive value. False positive results can be caused by heterozygote carriers, drug-induced hepatitis, nephrotic syndrome, acute viral hepatitis, alcoholic hepatitis, Menkes disease, chronic hepatitis, malabsorption, or excessive Zn intake.

An MRI of the brain can aid in the diagnosis of neurologic Wilson's.[2] Typical findings on T_1 sequences are hyperintensity in the lentiform nuclei and mesencephalic regions. T_2 hyperintensity is commonly seen in the basal ganglia – including the putamen, globus pallidus, and caudate nucleus – as well as the ventrolateral aspect of the thalamus.

Pharmacological treatment of Wilson's typically proceeds in two stages: removal of Cu accumulation and prevention of reaccumulation.[3] Removal of Cu accumulation is achieved with the use of Cu chelators such as D-penicillamine and trientine orally. Reaccumulation is prevented with oral Zn (increases endogenous chelators) or lower dose of D-penicillamine and trientine. A diet low in Cu-containing foods is also important in limiting disease progression. The foods highest in Cu include seafood, organ meats, whole grains, legumes, and chocolate.

Treatment of the complications of liver failure typically include diuresis, banding of esophageal varices and liver transplant for decompensated failure.[4] Treatment of tremor, parkinsonism, and psychiatric disturbance can improve quality of life for patients.

As noted above, there is a well-recognized phenomenon of neurologic worsening with initiation of chelator treatment.[4] Limited data show approximately a 10% incidence with D-penicillamine. There is some evidence that trientine has significantly lower risk from case reports. There is a theoretical lower risk with combined chelator and Zn therapy. Guidelines are to monitor for neurologic worsening after initiation of chelator treatment and if it is suspected to discontinue D-penicillamine and switch to trientine and/or Zn.

Untreated Wilson's disease is fatal; however, the prognosis for patients with appropriate treatment is excellent, with the majority of neurologic, hepatic, and psychiatric manifestations resolving over time as Cu is removed from the body.[3] In countries with well-developed healthcare systems, Wilson's is increasingly diagnosed early in the disease course and as a result tends to be managed aggressively and result in less death and disability.

The case presented gives an example of Wilson's disease which had been left largely untreated. Mrs. A's disease led to tremor, dysarthria, reduced coordination, liver cirrhosis, short-term memory impairment and Kayser-Fleischer rings and overall significant disability. Although presentations like these are increasingly rare, clinicians should stay vigilant in situations of unexplained hepatic or neurological dysfunction, especially when seen together, to catch this treatable disease early.

References

1. DiDonato M, Bibudhendra S. Copper transport and its alterations in Menkes and Wilson diseases. *BBA Mol Basis Dis.* 1997;1360(1):3–16.

2. Lorincz MT. Neurologic Wilson's disease. *Ann NY Acad Sci.* 2010;1184(1):173–187.

3. Roberts EA, Michael LS. Diagnosis and treatment of Wilson disease: an update. *Hepatology.* 2008;47(6):2089–2111.

4. European Association for the Study of the Liver. EASL clinical practice guidelines: Wilson's disease. *J Hepatol.* 2012;56(3):671–685.

5. Kitzberger R, Madl C, Ferenci P. Wilson's disease. *Metab Brain Dis.* 2005;20:295.

Tremor, Hallucinations, and Cognitive Decline

Philippe Huot, Antoine Duquette, and Michel Panisset

24.1 Clinical History – Main Complaint

A 72-year-old woman was seen with her husband at the movement disorder clinic. She was referred by her attending neurologist who has been following her for 9 years for Parkinson's disease (PD). Her symptoms had begun 10 years ago, with a left arm tremor that progressively worsened to affect the left side of her body and her right arm. The tremor was accompanied by generalized slowness of movement and stiffness. She was put on L-3,4-dihydroxyphenylalanine (L-DOPA) 8 years ago with a good initial response. Doses were progressively increased over the years. When seen at the clinic, she was taking L-DOPA/carbidopa (referred to as L-DOPA) 100/25 mg 1.5 pills every 3 hours from 6:00 a.m. to midnight, a total of 10.5 pills daily. Sometimes, she had to take an extra pill at night because of difficulty turning over in bed. She believed the effect of the antiparkinsonian medication was not lasting more than 2.5 hours and felt uncomfortable, with tremor resurgence, about 30 min before taking the next L-DOPA dose. Approximately 1 hour after L-DOPA intake, she would present fidgetiness and mild abnormal movements that were not bothersome but that were noticed by her husband and children. She had a few accidental falls. She sometimes experienced dizziness upon standing up rapidly. Approximately 1 year ago, she began experiencing visual hallucinations (VHs) that were, at times, frightening and prevented the neurologist from increasing L-DOPA doses. Most of the times, the VHs consisted of bugs, but on a few occasions they encompassed faces of unknown people. She had to be put on quetiapine 25 mg a.m. and 50 mg at bedtime to alleviate these VHs. Her husband was also concerned that she had become more forgetful in the past year. She was more apathetic and was not interested in going out anymore. At times, she was going through episodes of confusion. She was also experiencing episodes of daytime sleepiness and would have to nap for at least 1 hour every afternoon.

24.2 General History

The patient was a right-handed retired nurse. She was living with her husband in an apartment. The couple had two children, both of whom were in their 40s and in good health. She quit smoking 35 years ago. She drank one glass of wine per week. She had never used recreational drugs. Her past medical history was significant for hypothyroidism and hypertension, for which she was taking L-thyroxin and an angiotensin-converting enzyme inhibitor.

24.3 Family History

The patient's family history was negative for neurological and psychiatric disorders. Her mother died at 93 years from a myocardial infarction, while her father died at 92 from a pulmonary embolism. She had one brother, who was 70 and suffered from diabetes mellitus type 2 and hypertension.

24.4 General Examination

The patient was seen in the afternoon. She had taken three doses of L-DOPA (1.5 pills of 100/25 mg L-DOPA/carbidopa), the last one an hour ago. She was seen while in the "on" state.

Blood pressure when lying flat was 120/75, pulse 70/min. Standing blood pressure, 5 minutes later, was 115/50, pulse 74/min.

General neurological examination revealed saccadic smooth pursuits with mild upward gaze limitation. Blinking rate was reduced. There was mild hypomimia. Speech was soft and monotonous. Cranial nerves were otherwise unremarkable. There were no square-wave jerks. Deep tendon reflexes were normal and symmetrical. Plantar response was flexor bilaterally. Muscle strength was normal. Vibration and light touch were normal. There was no cerebellar anomaly.

The patient exhibited mild left arm and leg tremor at rest. Tremor was reemerging upon maintaining a posture for a few seconds. There was no kinetic tremor. There was mild bradykinesia that affected both the upper and lower limbs but was more pronounced on the left side. Muscle tone was increased in the neck and the four extremities, slightly more on the left than on the right side. Mild choreic dyskinesia affecting both lower extremities was seen when the patient was concentrating. Gait was slow, with reduced left arm swing, but there was no shuffling.

109

Turns were decomposed. Pull test showed a loss of postural reflexes.

Montreal Cognitive Assessment (MoCA) score was 17/30. Attention and concentration were relatively preserved, as the patient performed well at the tapping, serial subtraction, and digit span tasks. Language was mildly impaired; she confounded the rhinoceros with a hippopotamus. Repetition was intact. She was oriented to time and place. Executive functions were also impaired, as she could not complete the trail-making test, could not name more than seven words starting with the letter "F," and had difficulty with the verbal abstraction task. She was unable to recall the five words without cue. She had visuospatial impairment, as she could not successfully copy a cube and draw a clock.

She did not report any hallucinations during the questionnaire or the physical examination.

24.5 Special Studies

Routine biochemical and hematological test results were normal. A magnetic resonance imaging (MRI) of the brain was normal for the patient's age. A $[^{18}F]$-fluorodeoxyglucose (FDG) positron emission tomography (PET) revealed hypometabolism in the parietal and occipital areas, as can be seen in cases of PD with dementia. Electroencephalogram (EEG) was normal.

24.6 Diagnosis

The clinical picture of the patient was evocative of idiopathic PD, which consists of bradykinesia and at least one of tremor, rigidity, and/or postural instability.[1] Unilateral onset, disease duration, and response to dopamine replacement therapy also argued for PD and made other parkinsonian disorders unlikely. For instance, in diffuse Lewy body disease, the cognitive and psychiatric manifestations appear earlier in the disease process than in the present case. The patient experienced motor complications, that is, L-DOPA-induced dyskinesia and motor fluctuations, as well as non-motor complications, that is, orthostatic hypotension, VHs, apathy, and cognitive impairment.

24.7 Follow-Up

The patient's medication was adjusted in a stepwise fashion to minimize adverse effects due to rapid drug changes. Orthostatic hypotension was successfully treated by adding domperidone 5 mg three times daily. Entacapone was tried and discontinued rapidly because of dyskinesia exacerbation. Whereas amantadine might have alleviated dyskinesia, its anticholinergic action and potential deleterious effect on cognition prevented its use. Because of her age and cognitive deficits, the patient was not a candidate for deep-brain stimulation surgery. Her caregiver refused the option of intra-jejunal L-DOPA infusion.

A trial of rasagiline was undertaken. Rasagiline 1 mg daily diminished the end-of-dose loss of L-DOPA anti-parkinsonian action she was experiencing 30 min before the next dose was due. However, rasagiline increased severity of the VHs. To alleviate these, quetiapine was increased to 75 mg twice daily, which led to excessive daytime sleepiness. Quetiapine was replaced by clozapine 12.5 mg at bedtime, after which the VHs disappeared. The addition of clozapine also resulted in reduced dyskinesia severity. The patient is now undergoing regular complete blood counts, to monitor white blood cells, as clozapine can cause agranulocytosis in approximately 1% of users. The next step was to treat the patient's cognitive impairment. To that end, rivastigmine 4.6 mg daily was prescribed as a transdermal patch. It was well tolerated and was increased to 9.5 mg daily 1 month later.

The patient was seen 4 months after the last adjustments were made. She was then taking L-DOPA, rasagiline, domperidone, clozapine, and rivastigmine. She was presenting motor fluctuations at times, not regularly. Orthostatic hypotension had not resumed. She had not experienced VHs, and she and her husband believed that she was more alert and less forgetful. MoCA score was 22.

24.8 Discussion

PD is the second most common neurodegenerative disorder and affects 1% of the population above 60 - years old and 4% above 80.[2] With disease progression and chronic dopamine replacement therapy, patients develop motor and non-motor complications. According to the Sydney Multicentre Study of Parkinson's disease,[3] L-DOPA-induced dyskinesia affects as many as 95% of patients after 15 years of dopaminergic therapy, while motor fluctuations affect 96% of patients. Psychosis and VHs are encountered in as many as 50% of patients. Whereas dementia is encountered in 48% of patients, cognitive decline is present in as many as 84% of patients at that time.

VHs are the most common manifestation of PD psychosis, and are also the most prevalent form of hallucinations in PD, although auditory, olfactory, and tactile hallucinations are also encountered. The phenomenology of VHs is broad, ranging from shadows at the periphery of visual fields to well-formed VHs of animals and faces. According to the International Parkinson and Movement Disorder Society (IPMDS) evidence-based medicine (EBM) review on the treatment of non-motor symptoms of PD published in 2011, clozapine is efficacious at reducing psychosis and VHs.[4] However, because of the risk of agranulocytosis associated with its use, clozapine is often prescribed after trials of quetiapine have proven ineffective, despite the fact that quetiapine has not been conclusively shown to be effective in alleviating PD psychosis. Recently, pimavanserin was marketed in the United States for the specific indication of PD psychosis. Pimavanserin was effective at reducing PD psychosis in a Phase III clinical trial.

Cognitive impairment in PD affects a breadth of cognitive processes encompassing attentional, executive, language, and memory, as well as visuospatial functions.[5] According to the IPMDS EBM review on the treatment of non-motor symptoms of PD,

rivastigmine is efficacious to enhance cognitive functions in PD dementia.[4]

24.9 Take-Home Messages

Advanced PD is characterized by a breadth of motor and non-motor complications that can significantly impair patients' quality of life. Non-motor complications are increasingly recognized as a major problem in advanced PD. Psychosis and VHs, as well as cognitive decline and dementia, are deemed more burdensome than motor complications in late PD. They also are a major reason for institutionalization. Because treatments are available that can alleviate them, it is important to be aware of the issue of non-motor complications when caring for patients with advanced PD.

Financial Disclosure

There are no financial disclosures relevant to this manuscript and no conflict of interest.

Acknowledgments

The present work was supported by Université de Montréal and Centre Hospitalier de l'Université de Montréal.

References

1. Hughes AJ, Daniel SE, Kilford L, Lees AJ. Accuracy of clinical diagnosis of idiopathic Parkinson's disease: a clinico-pathological study of 100 cases. *J Neurol Neurosurg Psychiatry.* 1992;55(3):181–184.

2. de Lau LM, Breteler MM. Epidemiology of Parkinson's disease. *Lancet Neurol.* 2006;5 (6):525–535.

3. Hely MA, Morris JG, Reid WG, Trafficante R. Sydney Multicenter Study of Parkinson's disease: non-L-dopa-responsive problems dominate at 15 years. *Mov Disord.* 2005;20(2):190–199.

4. Seppi K, Weintraub D, Coelho M, et al. The Movement Disorder Society Evidence-Based Medicine Review Update: treatments for the non-motor symptoms of Parkinson's disease. *Mov Disord.* 2011;26 (Suppl 3):S42–S80.

5. Weintraub D, Burn DJ. Parkinson's disease: the quintessential neuropsychiatric disorder. *Mov Disord.* 2011;26 (6):1022–1031.

Dementia Following Stroke

Laksanun Cheewakriengkrai and Bandit Sirilert

25.1 Clinical History – Main Complaint

An 83-year-old, right-handed woman with behavioral changes for 2 days was seen at the neurology outpatient clinic of Phramongkutklao hospital.

25.2 General History

Twelve days prior to the visit, the patient was manifesting behavioral and personality changes, which can be characterized by irritability, talkativeness, and paranoia. She had false beliefs that her grandchildren and neighbors burglarized her home and that her brother stole her land. Furthermore, her recent memory had declined. She repeated questions and was unable to remember the meals that she had eaten and where she placed things.

Ten days earlier, her symptoms were getting worse. Her mood became more aggressive. She had difficulty in some routine functions, such as grocery shopping; she lost interest in cooking, which she used to enjoy doing. Her basic daily living activities remained unremarkable. No headache, fever, motor weakness, speech problem, ataxia, or hallucination was observed. She denied medical illness in the past. She had no history of smoking, drinking, or using any medication. Her education level was primary school. The patient visited a private hospital and was referred to Phramongkutklao hospital.

25.3 Family History

Her parents passed away when she was young. She has an elder sister who was diagnosed with ischemic stroke at the age of 60. The patient has three children who are healthy. No family history of neurodegenerative or psychiatric problems is known.

25.4 Examination

She was alert and cooperative during the examination, but appeared to be irritable and angry in mood. Vital signs showed regular pulse rate of 90 bpm and blood pressure of 110/60 mmHg. Physical examination was unremarkable, including the cardiovascular system. Neurological examination revealed normal cranial nerves. In the motor examination, the patient had no abnormal movement, posture, or fasciculation. Her tone was normal. She had full proximal and distal strength: 5/5 throughout all four extremities. No cortical lobe signs, frontal lobe releasing signs, or neglect was observed. Sensory examination was intact position, vibration, and pinprick sensation. The reflexes were 2+ and symmetrical with no evidence of clonus. Plantar responses were flexor. Coordination examination was intact with no evidence of dysdiadokinesis, intention tremor, heel-to–knee, or positive rebound. Her gait was normal and the Rhomberg test was unremarkable.

On the Montreal Cognitive Assessment (MoCA) she scored 8/30. She lost five points in executive/visuospatial; two points in naming, number "1" tapping test, and letter fluency; three points in calculation; five points in delayed recall; and five points in orientation. On the Geriatric Depression Scale (GDS), the patient scored 2/15. This demonstrated that she did not have depression. Clinical dementia rating (CDR) scale was evaluated and her rating was 1. On the Instrumental Activities of Daily Living (IADL) Questionnaire with score range 0–8, where a lower score indicates a higher level of dependence, she scored 1.

25.5 Special Studies

Routine blood tests were done. Most of them were negative, except for complete blood count, which showed Hb 14.2 g/dL, Hct 45.1%, WBC 11,600 /uL, PMN 72%, lymphocyte 20%, monocyte 3%, eosinophil 2%, basophil 3%, and platelet 623,000 /uL. Peripheral blood smear confirmed thrombocytosis: platelet counts were 30–40 per oil field. Investigations were done and found positive for *JAK2 V617F* gene mutation. Electrocardiogram (EKG) demonstrated normal sinus rhythm. Magnetic resonance imaging (MRI) and magnetic resonance angiography (MRA) of the brain showed restricted diffusion in diffuse weight imaging at the left temporo-occipital and thalamus. MRA showed focal stenosis of the left posterior cerebral artery. Internal carotid arteries, middle cerebral arteries, and anterior cerebral arteries were normal (Figure 25.1).

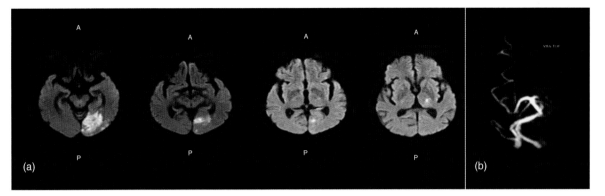

Figure 25.1 Imaging study that shows (a) restricted diffusion at the left temporo-occipital and thalamus (b) focal stenosis of left posterior cerebral artery.

25.6 Diagnosis

The provisional diagnosis was vascular dementia, strategic infarction subtype, based on the combination of acute behavioral changes, cognitive decline, and MRI findings compatible with acute cerebral infarction at the left thalamus. In general, the common causes of stroke are cardioembolic, athero-thrombotic, and lacunar infarction. However, the etiology of stroke in our patient was explained by essential thrombocytosis (ET) from the *JAK2 V617F* gene mutation, which has been infrequently reported.

Essential thrombocytosis is a chronic myeloproliferative disorder in which clonal hematopoietic stem cell disorder causes an abnormal increase in the amount of megakaryocytes, which results in an increase in the amount of platelets produced. The concomitant thrombotic events include abnormalities in macrovascular circulation, such as cerebrovascular, coronary, and peripheral arterial disease, and in microvascular circulation, such as erythromelalgia, ocular migraine, and transient ischemic attack (TIA). In a study of 1,099 first-stroke patients, essential thrombocythemia is associated with ischemic stroke in 0.54% of the cases.[1] This group accounted for 42.8% of all hematologic disorders associated with ischemic stroke and represented 12.5% of the patients diagnosed with essential thrombocythemia during the study period.

25.7 Follow-Up

The patient has been followed up every 3 months. Atypical antipsychotic and antiplatelet drugs along with donepezil were given to control her symptoms.

However, low performance in activities of daily living, delusion, and aggressive behaviors remained persistent. Thrombocytosis is well controlled by hydroxyurea.

25.8 Discussion

Vascular dementia (VaD) is the second most common cause of dementia, after Alzheimer's disease. It is recognized by a slow, progressive decline in cognitive functions, which can occur in a stepwise manner.[2] The symptoms are related to cerebrovascular disease (CVD) which is evident from the presence of focal signs on neurological examination and relevant CVD on brain imaging. The pathogenesis ranges from vascular occlusion to hemorrhages, whose causes can be atherosclerotic, embolic, hypoperfusion, and hereditary, such as in CADASIL (cerebral autosomal-dominant arteriopathy with subcortical infarcts and leukoencephalopathy). Several evidences indicate that the pathologies of vascular dementia and AD often coexist, especially in older patients with dementia.

Vascular dementia encompasses a wide spectrum of disorders. The National Institute of Neurological Disorders and Stroke – Canadian Stroke Network (NINDS-CSN) proposed the term vascular cognitive impairment (VCI) to cover the wide variety of syndromes.[3] This term ranges in intensity from mild cognitive impairment to full-blown dementia and in presentation of various cognitive disorders. Examples include vascular mild cognitive impairment, post-stroke dementia, multi-infarct dementia, subcortical ischemic vascular disease, strategic infarct; anterior cerebral artery infarct, parietal lobe infarcts, thalamic infarction, cingulate gyrus infarction, hypoperfusion dementia, hemorrhagic dementia, dementia caused by specific arteriopathies, and mixed AD with vascular dementia. VCI is being used more widely by physicians. Nevertheless, it has sometimes been misinterpreted as mild cognitive impairment (MCI) due to vascular factors. Later on, vascular cognitive disorder (VCD) has been proposed, with categories of mild VCD and major VCD.[4] This is a continuum from normal functioning to dementia, which is similar to cognitive disorders in other etiologies. The concept of VCD has been adopted in the *Diagnostic and Statistical Manual of Mental Disorders* (*DSM-5*) using the terms mild and major neurocognitive disorders, based on whether they interfere with independence in everyday activities or not.[5] The diagnosis criteria for major neurocognitive disorders are presented in Table 25.1.

Signs and symptoms in dementia after cerebrovascular disease can vary widely, depending on the severity of the blood vessel damage and the part of the brain affected. Mostly, executive functions are more affected rather than memory, which is typical in Alzheimer's disease.

Disinhibition, apathy, and akinetic mutism are typically present in early stage, if the prefrontal-subcortical circuits are interrupted. Imaging study is also important to support the diagnosis and differentiate other causes of dementia. Besides MRI which showed vascular lesion related with symptoms, functional imaging, such as positron emission tomography, may be useful for differentiating vascular dementia from AD. Hypoperfusion and hypometabolism can be observed in the frontal lobe, including the cingulate and superior frontal gyri, in patients with vascular dementia, whereas a reduction in parieto-temporal cortex, posterior cingulate, and precuneus pattern is observed in early AD patients.[6]

Management of vascular dementia should focus on preventing vascular risk factors and comorbidities. Cholinesterase inhibitors and **N-Methyl-D-aspartate receptor antagonists**, which are licensed and well-recognized drugs for AD, are used in vascular dementia based on suggestive evidence showing neuropathological and neurochemical overlap between the two disorders, in particular, the suggestion of cholinergic deficit in vascular dementia. However, a meta-analysis of randomized controlled trials showed only small benefits on cognitive outcomes, while the

Table 25.1 *DSM-5* criteria for major vascular neurocognitive disorders

A. Evidence of significant cognitive decline from a previous level of performance in one or more cognitive domains:

Learning and memory

Language

Executive function

Complex attention

Perceptual-motor

Social cognition

B. The cognitive deficits interfere with independence in everyday activities. At a minimum, assistance should be required with complex instrumental activities of daily living, such as paying bills or managing medications.

C. The cognitive deficits do not occur exclusively in the context of a delirium.

D. The cognitive deficits are not better explained by another mental disorder (major depressive disorder, schizophrenia).

E. The clinical features are consistent with a vascular etiology, as suggested by either of the following:

Onset of the cognitive deficits is temporally related to one or more cerebrovascular events.

Evidence for decline is prominent in complex attention (including processing speed) and frontal-executive function.

F. There is evidence of the presence of cerebrovascular disease from history, physical examination, and/or neuroimaging considered sufficient to account for the neurocognitive deficits.

G. The deficits are not better explained by another brain disease or systemic disorder.

benefits on global functioning, activities of daily living, and behaviors have not been consistently reported.[7] As for cerebrolysin, a peptide purified from pig brain proteins, there have been some reports of positive trials, which showed improvements in cognitive function and global function in patients with VaD of mild-to-moderate severity. But, due to the limited number of included trials (six trials were pooled), varying treatment durations, and short-term follow-up, there is insufficient evidence to recommend cerebrolysin as a routine treatment for patients with VaD.[8] Finally, non-pharmacological management of noncognitive symptoms, appropriate psychosocial, and other support are beneficial to improve the quality of life of the patients and caregivers.[9]

References

1. Arboix A, Besses C, Acín P, et al. Ischemic stroke as first manifestation of essential thrombocythemia. Report of six cases. *Stroke.* 1995;26 (8):1463–1466.

2. Roman GC, Tatemichi TK, Erkinjuntti T, et al. Vascular dementia: diagnostic criteria for research studies. Report of the NINDS-AIREN International Workshop. *Neurology.* 1993;43 (2):250–260.

3. O'Brien JT, Erkinjuntti T, Reisberg B, et al. Vascular cognitive impairment. *Lancet Neurol.* 2003;2(2): 89–98.

4. Sachdev P, Kalaria R, O'Brien J, et al. Diagnostic criteria for vascular cognitive disorders: a VASCOG statement. *Alzheimer Dis Assoc Disord.* 2014;28 (3):206–218.

5. American Psychiatric Association. *Diagnostic and Statistical Manual of Mental Disorders (DSM 5).* Washington, DC: American Psychiatric Association; 2013.

6. Ishii K. PET approaches for diagnosis of dementia. *AJNR Am J Neuroradiol.* 2014;35 (11):2030–2038.

7. Kavirajan H, Schneider LS. Efficacy and adverse effects of cholinesterase inhibitors and memantine in vascular dementia: a meta-analysis of randomised controlled trials. *Lancet Neurol.* 2007;6(9):782–792.

8. Chen N, Yang M, Guo J, et al. Cerebrolysin for vascular dementia. *Cochrane Database Syst. Rev.* 2013;31(1):CD008900.

9. O'Brien JT, Thomas A. Vascular dementia. *Lancet.* 2015;386 (10004):1698–1706.

Vascular Cognitive Impairment

Kok Pin Ng and Nagaendran Kandiah

26.1 Case Presentation

An 85-year-old woman with hypertension and hyperlipidemia presented with gradual and progressive cognitive impairment for more than 2 years, involving cognitive domains of memory, executive function, visuospatial and mood. She has short-term memory loss such as forgetting whether she has eaten or showered. She will also ask the same questions repeatedly. However, her long-term memory remains intact. She has forgotten how to cook and has recently burnt the pot while cooking on the stove. She is also unable to manage finances and often gives the wrong change while buying her usual groceries. She has lost her way a few times in places where she is familiar with. In addition, she started having mood swings, low mood, and poor sleep. Physical examination reveals mild bilateral bradykinesia, absence of postural or rest tremors, normal limb power, tone and tendon reflexes. She has lower limb apraxia and mild postural instability. Her Mini-Mental State Examination (MMSE) was 16. While she scored 0 for delayed recall, she was able to recall all 3 objects with either category or lexical cueing.

Her brain magnetic resonance imaging (MRI) shows confluent periventricular and deep white matter T2 hyperintensities, chronic tiny infarcts in the left lentiform nucleus and pons, and chronic microhemorrhages in the left thalamus and right pons. While there are global involutional changes, there is no disproportionate hippocampal atrophy (Figure 26.1). She is diagnosed with moderate dementia, due to vascular dementia and concomitant Alzheimer's disease (AD). She is treated with cholinesterase inhibitors and her cardiovascular risk factors are optimized.

26.2 Discussion

This case illustrates a patient with cerebrovascular risk factors, who presents with gradual and progressive decline in cognition, mainly affecting her executive function, visuospatial, and mood/behavior cognitive domains. While she had short-term memory loss, this improved when given cues. Her MRI brain shows extensive small vessel cerebrovascular disease (CVD).

Vascular cognitive impairment (VCI), which encompasses all forms of cognitive impairment with CVD contributing to the symptoms, is the second most common cause of dementia after AD. VCI makes up 10–20% of dementia in North America and Europe, and in a longitudinal, population-based study looking at the pathological correlates of dementia, the estimates of adjusted population attributable risk of dementia due to cerebral microinfarcts is 33%. VCI also often coexists with other neurodegenerative pathologies, such as Alzheimer's pathology. From our Asian cohorts, we found that 28.3% of mild AD and 39.7% of moderate-severe AD have severe white matter hyperintensities (WMH).

26.2.1 Diagnostic Criteria for VCI

There are a number of clinical diagnostic criteria for VCI. The Hachinski Ischemic Score (HIS) was first proposed to distinguish multi-infarct dementia from AD. Subsequent diagnostic criteria for VCI include the following:

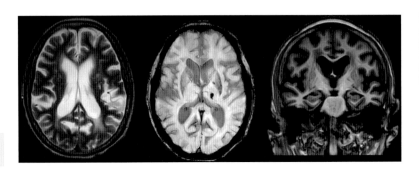

Figure 26.1 **MRI showing** confluent periventricular and deep white matter T2 hyperintensities, chronic tiny infarcts in the left lentiform nucleus and pons, and chronic microhemorrhages in the left thalamus and right pons.

1. International Classification of Diseases, Tenth Revision (ICD-10)
2. National Institute of Neurological Disorders and Stroke-Association Internationale pour la Recherche et l'Enseignement en Neurosciences (NINDS-AIREN)
3. State of California Alzheimer's Disease Diagnostic and Treatment Centers (ADDTC)
4. American Heart Association/American Stroke Association (AHA/ASA)[1]
5. International Society of Vascular Behavioural and Cognitive Disorders (Vas-Cog)[2]
6. Diagnostic and Statistical Manual of Mental Disorders, Fifth Edition (*DSM-5*)

These criteria require cognitive impairment to be present together with evidence of a contribution of CVD to the symptoms, supported by clinical history, physical examination, neuropsychological assessment, and neuroimaging. While the NINDS-AIREN and ADDTC require the presence of memory impairment as one of the criteria, the AHA/ASA, Vas-Cog, and *DSM-5* allow a decline in any of the cognitive domains.

The AHA/ASA, Vas-Cog, and *DSM-5* also acknowledge that VCI may present as poststroke VCI or nonstroke forms of VCI, such as that caused by subcortical ischemic disease. In this regard, neuroimaging and neuropathology studies play an important role in identifying CVD associated with cognitive impairment in individuals who do not present with a clinical history of stroke.

26.2.2 Vascular Pathology of VCI

The Vas-Cog criteria have subclassified VCI according to the underlying cerebrovascular pathology:[2]

1. Parenchymal Lesions of Vascular Etiology (large vessel atherothromboembolic disease, small vessel disease, hemorrhage, hypoperfusion)
2. Types of Vascular Pathologies (atherosclerosis, cardiac, atherosclerotic, and systemic emboli, arteriolosclerosis, lipohyalinosis, cerebral amyloid angiopathy, vasculitis, venous collagenosis, arteriovenous fistulae, hereditary angiopathies (e.g., cerebral autosomal dominant arteriopathy with subcortical infarcts and leukoencephalopathy [CADASIL]), berry aneurysms, miscellaneous vasculopathies (e.g., moyamoya disease), and cerebral venous thrombosis)

26.2.3 Clinical Presentation

In VCI, the clinical presentation is dependent on the location of the predominant CVD pathology.

If the pathology involves acute lesions in the cortical region, patients may present with a clinical stroke, resulting in a sudden onset, and stepwise deterioration. Cognitive impairment is specific to the cortical regions affected. In the medial frontal region, symptoms include executive dysfunction, abulia, or apathy. In the parietal region, symptoms include aphasia, apraxia, agnosia, neglect, and visuospatial and constructional difficulty. In the medial temporal region, symptoms include anterograde amnesia.

If the pathology such as lacunar infarction and chronic microvascular ischemia affect the deep cerebral nuclei and white matter pathways in the subcortical region, this leads to a disruption of the frontal-subcortical circuits. Typical symptoms include focal motor signs; gait disturbance; unsteadiness and frequent, unprovoked falls; mood and behavioral changes; abulia; apathy; depression; emotional incontinence; and cognitive impairment characterized by a relatively mild memory decline, slowed processing speed, and executive dysfunction. The course of subcortical VCI may be either gradual or stepwise.

26.2.4 Cognitive Profiles of VCI

VCI is associated with greater impairments in executive function and processing speed and relatively lesser impairment in episodic memory. On the other hand, AD is most often associated with episodic memory impairment before other cognitive domains become impaired. It is also important to note that some degree of memory impairment is present in VCI.

26.2.5 Evaluating Cerebrovascular Disease in VCI

The presence of CVD in VCI may be established based on clinical history, physical examination, and neuroimaging.

For the diagnosis of poststroke VCI, a clinical history of stroke supported by neuroimaging evidence of acute infarction or hemorrhage consistent with patient's presentation is required. In addition, the patient should be cognitively intact prior to the stroke followed by an acute onset of cognitive impairment after the stroke. In this regard, questionnaires such as the Informant Questionnaire on Cognitive Decline in the Elderly (IQCODE) may be used to assess for prestroke cognitive decline.

When there is no history of an acute stroke, neuroimaging such as MRI/CT plays an important role in identifying silent infarcts or small vessel CVD including white matter hyperintensities, perivascular space, and cerebral microbleeds (Figure 26.2). The presence of cardiovascular risk factors and clinical symptoms of executive dysfunction, slowed processing speed, gait disturbance, and mood and behavioral changes can further support a diagnosis of subcortical VCI.

26.2.6 Associations of Small Vessel Cerebrovascular Disease and Dementia

Population-based studies show that silent infarcts and white matter hyperintensities predict dementia while postmortem studies further show that small vessel CVD such as small infarcts, independently predicts dementia risk. Higher numbers of infarcts and higher volumes of white matter hyperintensities are also associated with higher risk of cognitive impairment.

26.2.7 Management

The management of VCI can be both pharmacological or non-pharmacological.

Given that cholinergic dysfunction has been shown in VCI, the role of acetylcholinesterase inhibitors in VCI has been studied in clinical trials. A meta-analysis of six cholinesterase inhibitor trials (three donepezil, two galantamine, one rivastigmine) which were of 6-month duration and had similar vascular dementia criteria and outcome measures found an overall statistically significant cognitive benefit as measured using the ADAS-COG scale change from baseline.[3] However, there is no consistent benefit using measures of global impression of change outcomes. Hence, it is concluded that cholinesterase inhibitors produce small benefits in cognition of uncertain clinical significance in patients with mild to moderate vascular dementia. While there is insufficient evidence to recommend acetylcholinesterase inhibitors for patients with pure VCI, they are often prescribed in part because of the known co-association of VCI and AD.

Memantine is a N-Methyl-D-aspartate receptor antagonist that is often used in combination with an acetylcholinesterase inhibitor in patients with AD and

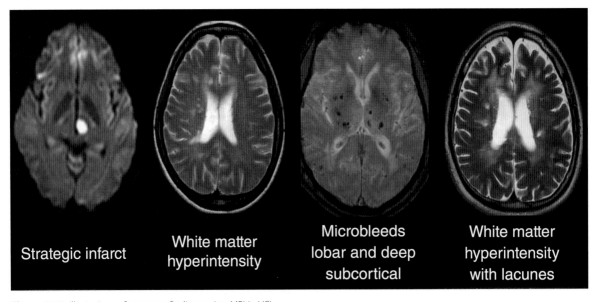

| Strategic infarct | White matter hyperintensity | Microbleeds lobar and deep subcortical | White matter hyperintensity with lacunes |

Figure 26.2 Illustrations of common findings using MRI in VCI.

VCI. However, the demonstrated benefits of memantine are not well established, and the duration of the trials was short at 28 weeks.

One of the most important components in managing VCI is the identification and optimization of the causative cerebrovascular risk factors for secondary prevention of progression or recurrence of an acute cerebrovascular event. In poststroke VCI, recurrence of stroke is a strong risk factor for worsening of cognitive function and dementia[4] and with adequate control of cerebrovascular risk factors, it may be possible to slow down the progression of VCI.

Patients with cognitive impairment and clinical or radiologic evidence of cerebrovascular lesions should be screened and treated for vascular risk factors, especially hypertension. A consensus-based scientific review by the American Heart Association/American Stroke Association (AHA/ASA) states that blood pressure lowering to lower the risk of poststroke dementia is effective and that it is recommended to lower blood pressure in people at risk for VCI.[1] In people at risk for VCI, treatment of hyperglycemia and hypercholesterolemia may be reasonable.[1]

There is increasing evidence showing that modifiable health behaviors such as smoking, alcohol intake, physical activity, and diet are associated with cognitive function. In a study looking at health behaviors from early to late midlife over a 17-year period as predictors of cognitive function, both the number of unhealthy behaviors and their duration are associated with subsequent impairment in executive function and memory in later life.[5] Multimodality interventions to improve population control of cardiovascular risk factors further constitute a promising approach to prevent dementia. The Finnish Geriatric Intervention Study to Prevent Cognitive Impairment and Disability (FINGER) study which randomly assigned participants to a multidomain approach including cardiovascular risk factor control, diet, exercise, and cognitive training prevented decline in cognitive test scores.[6]

26.3 Conclusion

VCI represents the second most common cause of dementia and often coexists with AD pathophysiology. VCI may present as poststroke cognitive impairment or subcortical VCI due to small vessel CVD. Identification and optimization of the causative cerebrovascular risk factors plays an important role in the management of VCI.

References

1. Gorelick PB, Scuteri A, Black SE, et al. Vascular contributions to cognitive impairment and dementia: a statement for healthcare professionals from the American Heart Association/American Stroke Association. *Stroke*. 2011;42:2672–2713.

2. Sachdev P, Kalaria R, O'Brien J, et al. Diagnostic criteria for vascular cognitive disorders: a VASCOG statement. *Alzheimer Dis Assoc Disord*. 2014;28:206–218.

3. Kavirajan H, Schneider LS. Efficacy and adverse effects of cholinesterase inhibitors and memantine in vascular dementia: a meta-analysis of randomised controlled trials. *Lancet Neurol*. 2007;6:782–792.

4. Srikanth VK, Quinn SJ, Donnan GA, Saling MM, Thrift AG. Long-term cognitive transitions, rates of cognitive change, and predictors of incident dementia in a population-based first-ever stroke cohort. *Stroke*. 2006;37:2479–2483.

5. Sabia S, Nabi H, Kivimaki M, et al. Health behaviors from early to late midlife as predictors of cognitive function: the Whitehall II study. *Am J Epidemiol*. 2009;170:428–437. Accessed at: http://aje.oxfordjournals.org/cgi/content/long/170/4/428.

6. Ngandu T, Lehtisalo J, Solomon A, et al. A 2 year multidomain intervention of diet, exercise, cognitive training, and vascular risk monitoring versus control to prevent cognitive decline in at-risk elderly people (FINGER): a randomised controlled trial. *Lancet*. 2015;385:2255–2263.

Rapidly Progressive Behavioral Changes and Cognitive Symptoms in a 29-Year-Old Woman

Peter Hermann, Katharina Hein, Katrin Radenbach, and Inga Zerr

27.1 Case Report

27.1.1 Onset and Early Clinical Course

A 29-year-old woman was referred to a community hospital. She was accompanied by her parents. They reported that behavioral and personality changes had been present for 3 days. The patient suddenly had started to speak almost incomprehensibly. She also had become obtrusive and impulsive. In addition, she had talked to imaginary people and introduced herself as another person. The physicians at the hospital described her as an aggressive person with incoherent thinking, pathological crying, and hallucinations. No focal neurological signs were observed. With suspected schizophrenic psychosis, the patient was transferred to a psychiatric department.

Because of rapidly progressive symptoms, fluctuating vigilance, and mild leukocytosis in the blood, the patient was sent back to the casualty department the next day. A cerebral CT-scan showed no pathological results. A lumbar puncture was performed and the analysis of the cerebrospinal fluid (CSF) revealed elevated leukocyte count (36/μL). The patient was transferred to a general intensive care unit and received aciclovir 2,250 mg/d and ceftriaxon 2 g/d to treat the suspected infection of the central nervous system and haloperidol and diazepam because of the hallucinations and agitation. Another 2 days later, she was transferred to the neurological intensive care unit of a university hospital for further diagnosis and treatment.

27.1.2 Patient's Medical History

The patient had no personal or family history for psychiatric disorders. She did not misuse alcohol or illegal drugs. Before onset, she received no medication and no allergies or chronic internal diseases were present. She had normal intelligence and worked as an electronic technician until 3 days before onset of clinical symptoms. At the age of 13, she underwent a partial resection of the right ovary. Histopathological reports described a differentiated cystic teratoma (dermoid cyst), which showed no signs of malignity.

27.1.3 Imaging, EEG, and CSF-Analysis

A computed tomography (CT) scan 4 days after clinical onset showed no pathological results. The first cerebral magnetic resonance imaging (MRI) was performed 7 days after onset. Neuroradiologists described suspicious but not unambiguous signal hyperintensities of both hippocampi on fluid-attenuated inversion recovery (FLAIR)-weighted images (see Figure 27.1).

Several electroencephalographies (EEG) were performed during acute treatment but showed no distinct epileptiform activity. Depending on sedative medication, either massive movement artifacts or general slowing of normal rhythm were recorded. Later EEG showed rhythmic focal delta activity in frontal and temporal regions on both hemispheres.

The first lumbar puncture was performed 4 days after onset. Within a narrow time frame, an elevation of leucocytes (36/μL) as well as normal CSF proteins (430 mg/L), albumin ratio (4.9), lactate (1.8 mmol/L), and glucose could be measured. Because of the detection of intrathecal synthesis of IgG and pleocytosis, diagnosis of an inflammatory process of the brain was made. Specific antibodies against human herpes virus (HHV) 1-3, measles virus, rubella virus, Epstein–Barr virus, cytomegalovirus, and Borrelia were normal. Within 3 days after lumbar puncture, results from

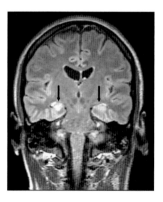

Figure 27.1 On T1 and DWI, no abnormalities and no pathological enhancement of contrast agent could be observed. Later MR-images showed the same results.

polymerase chain reaction (PCR) (HHV 1-3: negative) and detection of further antibodies were available. Paraneoplastic antibodies (e.g., GAD65, Ma1, Ma2, amphiphysin, Ri, Yo, HuD) were not detectable. Immunofluorescence for neuronal antibodies like CASPAR2, AMPAR1, AMPAR2, LGI1, and DPPX was negative but NMDA-receptor antibodies showed up clearly positive.

With history of ovarian teratoma in mind, abdominal imaging was performed. CT and MRI showed polycystic ovaries on both sides. Sonographically, a dermoid cyst of the right ovary was suspected.

27.1.4 Case Management and Further Course of Disease

When the patient had arrived at a specialized neurological intensive care unit, she was soporous. In addition, an acute renal failure with increased serum creatinine and decreased glomerual filtration rate was diagnosed. The differential diagnosis of the reduced vigilance might have been caused by a combination of sedative and antipsychotic medication, possible nonconvulsive seizures, or as direct consequence of encephalopathy or encephalitis. Antipsychotic medication was reduced and antiepileptic therapy with valproic acid was started, although the EEG showed no distinct epileptiform activity. The acute renal failure was most likely induced by previously started acyclovir therapy. Because of negative HHV-PCR, absence of bacterial growth in CSF cultures and history of ovarian teratoma, physicians suspected an autoimmune encephalitis. Then antiviral therapy was discontinued. In the further course, renal function recovered. Intravenous therapy with methylprednisolone (1 g/d) had already been induced 1 day before the patient was relocated. This therapy continued for overall 5 days. Meanwhile, the positive result for NMDA-receptor antibodies was available and plasmapheresis was planned. The patient had received three cycles, when a pneumonia occurred and had to be treated. Although abdominal CT and MRI showed no obvious results, recurrence of a right ovarian dermoid cyst was suspected sonographically. Plasmapheresis was discontinued for 1 week and the patient underwent a laparoscopic adnexectomy on the right side. Histopathological results showed a differentiated ovarian teratoma without signs of malignity. Plasmapheresis was continued for another four cycles. The patient became

more vigilant and showed less severe psychiatric symptoms. Oral medication with prednisolone was started. In follow-up CSF analysis, leucocyte count was decreasing.

The patient was discharged from intensive care unit and transferred to neurologic rehabilitation after 5 weeks of treatment. At this point, she was vigilant but still suffered from cognitive problems, especially severe memory deficits and psychomotor impairment. No major psychotic symptoms were present, but she still received haloperidol. During neurologic rehabilitation, an episode with agitation and hallucinations occurred and continued for 3 days. Antipsychotic medication was switched to olanzapine and the patient was transferred to a psychiatric ward, where no more aggressive behavior or psychotic symptoms were observed. However, cognitive deficits and depressive mood were still present. Medication with antidepressants was started and the patient could be relocated to complete neurological rehabilitation. Eight weeks after onset, the patient underwent another lumbar puncture as follow-up examination. As leucocyte count was normal and intrathecal IgG synthesis was not detectable anymore, slow reduction of prednisolone and valproic acid was started. However, NMDA-receptor antibody immunofluorescence was still slightly positive. Temporary reduction of olanzapine led to delusional mood without hallucination or agitation. Eight months after disease onset and after further outpatient treatment, the patient showed isolated moderate episodic memory deficits. Antipsychotic medication had been ceased. The patient still received lamotrigine and 7.5 mg prednisolone. For an overview, see Table 27.1, which summarizes CSF results, clinical symptoms, and most important therapeutic measures over a period of 8 months.

27.2 Discussion

We presented the case of a young woman with NMDA-receptor antibody positive limbic encephalitis, which was associated with a recurrent ovarian teratoma. On initial presentation, schizophrenic episode was suspected, but because of some less typical features, the CSF was investigated and paved the way for rapid diagnosis. Results of MRI were uncertain, which might be caused by previously induced steroid therapy. She received plasmapheresis and surgical treatment of the teratoma. Although having suffered

Table 27.1 Synopsis of symptoms, CSF-analysis, and treatment

Days after onset	Clinical symptoms	CSF				
		Cell count (/μL)	NMDA-R antibodies[a]			
			RC-IFT	IgA	IgG	IgM
0	Aggressiveness, derailment, delusions, incoherent speech, pathological crying, optical hallucination					
4	Same as above Fluctuating vigilance, sopor, complex focal seizures	36	Positive	1:320	1:320	1:1
→ Methylprednisolone, 1 g/d for 5 days						
10	Same as above	40	Positive	1:100	1:100	neg.
→ Plasmapheresis, 7 cycles → Oophorectomy → Oral prednisolone						
32	Incomplete orientation, memory, and psychomotor impairment	5	Positive	1:10	1:10	neg.
67	Impairment of episodic memory, mild psychotic symptoms after reduction of neuroleptic medication	1	Positive (slightly)			
156	Severe impairment of episodic memory	0		1:1	1:3	neg.
245	Moderate impairment of episodic memory	0				

[a] Results were received 3–5 days after lumbar puncture.

some medical complications, she fortunately recovered to a great extent.

Anti-NMDA receptor encephalitis is a rare disease, which was described first in 2007.[1] Affective and psychotic symptoms along with impaired episodic memory and seizures of temporal origin are major clinical features, most patients are female.[2] At primary clinical examination, the reported patient presented psychiatric symptoms which can easily mislead to diagnosis of schizophrenic psychosis. Impairment of episodic memory was evident in the later disease course but was probably masked by the other symptoms at onset. On the other hand, absent prodromal symptoms and no history of previous psychotic episodes should be suspicious for an organic disease. In this case, rapid progression of symptoms, autonomic dysregulation, elevated CSF leukocytes, and information of a previously diagnosed teratoma pointed to diagnosis of autoimmune paraneoplastic encephalitis. Anti-NMDA receptor encephalitis is associated with neoplasia in up to 80%, especially with teratoma in up to 60%.[3] Evidence for antibodies can be obtained using immunofluorescence technique on CSF. Testing CSF is obligate as NMDA receptor antibodies usually cannot be found in peripheral fluids.[4] The reported patient presented some other common paraclinical features (see Table 27.1). In patients with anti-NMDA receptor encephalitis, cerebral CT-scans are unremarkable but FLAIR- or T2-weighted MR images may show abnormal signal hyperintensities in the temporal cortex. Elevation of CSF leucocytes at early stages and decrease in the further course as well as evidence for intrathecal IgG synthesis are characteristic.[5] Predictive factors for a good outcome are the presence of surgically treatable neoplasia and an early start of therapy. Besides surgical measures, therapy should consist of high-dose steroid application and at least one additional immunologic therapy, for example, plasmapheresis or IVIG.[5] The patient received all recommended measures and showed only mild clinical residuals after 8 months. Such a good outcome has been described in up to 75% sufficiently treated patients.[2]

In conclusion, we emphasize the urgency of complete neurological workup including imaging and lumbar puncture in patients with acute onset and no prior history of psychotic symptoms. Early start of appropriate pharmacological and interventional therapy as well as surgical therapy of neoplasia can lead to a positive clinical outcome in patients with limbic encephalitis.

References

1. Sansing LH, Tüzün E, Ko MW, et al. A patient with encephalitis associated with NMDA receptor antibodies. *Nat Clin Pract Neurol.* 2007;3:291–296.

2. Dalmau J, Lancaster E, Martinez-Hernandez E, Rosenfeld MR, Balice-Gordon R. Clinical experience and laboratory investigations in patients with anti-NMDAR encephalitis. *Lancet Neurol.* 2011;10:63–74.

3. Tüzün E, Zhou L, Baehring JM, et al. Evidence for antibody-mediated pathogenesis in anti-NMDAR encephalitis associated with ovarian teratoma. *Acta Neuropathol.* 2009;118:737–743.

4. Prüss H, Dalmau J, Harms L, et al. Retrospective analysis of NMDA receptor antibodies in encephalitis of unknown origin. *Neurology.* 2010;75:1735–1739.

5. Irani SR, Bera K, Waters P, et al. N-methyl-D-aspartate antibody encephalitis: temporal progression of clinical and paraclinical observations in a predominantly non-paraneoplastic disorder of both sexes. *Brain.* 2010;133:1655–1667.

Young Woman Feeling Sick and Confused

Masamichi Ikawa, Akiko Matsunaga, and Makoto Yoneda

28.1 Clinical History

A 32-year-old right-handed woman developed persistent fever with malaise and nausea. The symptoms persisted for 2 weeks, after which she was admitted because of delirium, amnesia, and repetitive generalized convulsions with loss of consciousness. She had no remarkable past and family medical history, which included a history of abortions and thyroiditis. However, she had gained a body weight of 20 kg in the 1 year preceding this episode. She was not on medication and did not smoke or consume alcohol.

28.2 Examination

At admission, the patient had a body temperature of 37.2°C, blood pressure of 120/80 mmHg, pulse rate 70 beats per minute, regular respiratory rate of 12 breaths per minute, and oxygen saturation of 97% (room air). The patient's height was 167 cm, while the weight was 70 kg (body mass index: 25.1). The physical examination findings were unremarkable; we did not find edema in the extremities or enlargement of the thyroid gland. The patient was drowsy and in a state of confusion, along with amnesia. The function of the cranial nerves was intact. Muscular weakness, sensory disturbance, cerebellar ataxia, and involuntary movements were not observed. Tendon reflexes in the extremities were diminished without pathological reflex.

All routine laboratory data, including the white blood cell count (2,800/mL), serum sodium level (141 mEq/L), and CRP level (0.2 mg/dL) were normal. Although the patient was clinically euthyroid (TSH: 0.9 IU/mL, free T4: 1.2 ng/mL), both the antithyroid peroxidase (TPO) and anti-thyroglobulin (TG) antibodies were detected (57.5 IU/mL and 0.6 IU/mL, respectively; normal < 0.3 for both). Antibodies to nuclear (ANA), ds-DNA, Sm, and U1-RNP as well as C-ANCA and P-ANCA were not detected. Tumor marker test results for CA19–9 and CA125 were also negative. Cerebrospinal fluid (CSF) examination showed normal protein concentration (31 mg/dL) and no pleocytosis (1 cell/mL). DNA of herpes simplex virus 1 (HSV-1) and bacterial cultures were not detected. Lactate and pyruvate levels were normal

in both the serum and CSF samples. Electroencephalogram (EEG) revealed generalized slow waves with sporadic sharp waves. Brain MRI showed swelling with hyperintensities on fluid-attenuated inversion recovery (FLAIR) images in the bilateral medial temporal lobes and the insular cortices (Figure 28.1), suggesting limbic encephalitis. No obvious contrast-enhanced lesions were observed on the MRI. No tumors were identified on chest and abdominal CT images.

28.3 Special Studies

The symptoms and findings indicating encephalitis, such as persistent fever, psychosis, and dementia with seizures and abnormalities in the limbic areas on MR images, along with no evidence of infection suggested that the patient had a form of autoimmune limbic encephalitis (LE), particularly Hashimoto's encephalopathy (HE), because of the presence of antithyroid (TPO and TG) antibodies. Myxedema was excluded because the patient was euthyroid. Thus, we examined the serum for autoantibodies against the amino (NH$_2$)-terminal of α-enolase (NAE), a specific diagnostic marker of HE.[1] Immunoblotting of a recombinant NAE protein with the patient's serum sample showed a positive result for anti-NAE antibodies (titer, ×320) (Figure 28.2). In order to exclude other types of autoimmune limbic encephalitis, the serum sample was also tested for autoantibodies against the

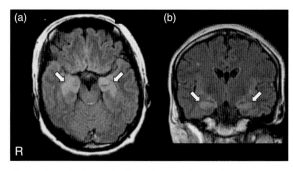

Figure 28.1 Brain MRI findings of the patient. FLAIR images show swelling with abnormal hyperintense signals in the bilateral medial temporal lobes (arrows), suggesting limbic encephalitis. Transverse (a) and sagittal images (b). R, right.

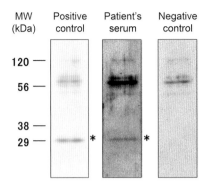

MW (kDa) | Positive control | Patient's serum | Negative control

120 —
56 —
38 —
29 — *

Figure 28.2 Immunoblotting of a recombinant NAE protein with the patient's serum. An NAE signal was detected at 29 kDa for the patient. *Position of the recombinant NAE. MW, molecular weight.

N-methyl-D-aspartate receptors (NMDAR), leucine-rich glioma inactivated 1 (LGI1), contactin-associated protein 2 (Caspr2), γ-aminobutyric acid-B receptor (GABA$_B$R), and α-amino-3-hydroxy-5-methylisoxazole-4-propionic acid receptor 1 and 2 (AMPAR1/2), none of which were detected in the serum. Paraneoplastic antibodies to Hu, Yo, and Ri were also not detected.

28.4 Diagnosis and Treatment

The patient was treated with methylprednisolone pulse therapy (1,000 mg for 3 days) followed by oral prednisolone (60 mg/day), in addition to sodium valproate. The patient showed good recovery, with mild residual disability including slight amnesia. The body weight spontaneously reduced after the treatment. No relapse has been observed during the follow-up period of more than 10 years.

The patient was diagnosed with HE based on the following diagnostic criteria:[2] neuropsychiatric symptoms, presence of antithyroid antibodies, and responsiveness to immunotherapy, in addition to the presence of anti-NAE antibodies. The neuropsychiatric symptoms and MRI findings that she presented with (i.e., psychosis and dementia with bilateral limbic lesions) as well as her favorable responsiveness to corticosteroid therapy suggest that the encephalopathy belongs to the category of an autoimmune LE. The possibility of LE associated with HSV-1 infection, systemic autoimmune diseases, and autoimmunity due to antibodies to the NMDAR, LGI1, Caspr2, GABA$_B$R, and anti-AMPAR1/2 were fully excluded.

Consequently, the final diagnosis of autoimmune LE associated with HE was made.

28.5 Discussion

HE is characterized as an autoimmune encephalopathy associated with antithyroid antibodies that shows a good response to immunotherapies, especially corticosteroids;[2] thus, HE is also called steroid-responsive encephalopathy associated with autoimmune thyroiditis (SREAT). The clinical entity and nosology have been debated because of the wide variety of clinical symptoms and the lack of diagnostic molecular markers of HE until recently. We recently performed proteomic analyses to identify a diagnostic marker of HE and discovered anti-NAE antibodies in the serum of patients with HE. These antibodies are highly specific for HE.[1]

Based on our study of 80 cases of HE, patients with HE typically present with acute neuropsychiatric symptoms (58%) such as amnesia, delirium, hallucination, and seizures, and occasionally, chronic dementia or psychosis (17%). In addition, HE includes various clinical subtypes resembling Creutzfeldt-Jakob disease (3%)[3] or cerebellar ataxia (16%).[4] In laboratory and radiological findings, most patients are in a euthyroid state, with antithyroid (TPO and/or TG) antibodies. CSF protein concentration is frequently increased (45%), with or without pleocytosis. Slow-wave activity is commonly observed on an EEG, occasionally with various paroxysmal epileptic discharges (80%). Although abnormalities on brain MRI are not commonly detected (36%), decreased regional cerebral blood flow is frequently observed on brain single-photon emission computed tomography (SPECT) (76%). Overall, the characteristic clinico-radiological features of HE are the highly frequent abnormalities on EEG and brain SPECT, in contrast to only mild organic changes on brain MRI, which indicates the reversibility of the disease by using appropriate immunotherapy in patients with HE.

Corticosteroids, such as oral prednisolone and methylprednisolone pulse therapy, are the first-line treatment for patients with HE. Most patients treated with corticosteroids show good recovery, but some patients (<20%) resist the treatment. In such cases, plasmapheresis or intravenous administration of immunoglobulin is considered as the second-line treatment. Since relapses of the symptoms often occur after tapering or discontinuing the corticosteroids, concomitant therapy with immunosuppressants is recommended.

The present case was diagnosed as autoimmune LE associated with HE. Recently, several autoantibodies against cell surface receptors or synaptic proteins, such as NMDAR, LGI1, Caspr2, $GABA_BR$, and AMPAR1/2, have been identified in patients with LE, in part associated with tumors. We recently reported another case of autoimmune LE with anti-NAE antibodies, diagnosed as HE similar to the present case.[5] These cases of LE associated with HE suggests that LE form, which commonly presents with psychosis and dementia, is another clinical subtype of HE.

In summary, HE often presents with neuropsychiatric symptoms similar to those seen in dementia, but is treatable by immunotherapies. Therefore, physicians must more attentively consider the possibility of HE as "treatable dementia", when they encounter a patient with atypical dementia and/or psychosis with the presence of antithyroid antibodies.

References

1. Yoneda M, Fujii A, Ito A, et al. High prevalence of serum autoantibodies against the amino terminal of alpha-enolase in Hashimoto's encephalopathy. *J Neuroimmunol.* 2007;185:195–200.

2. Shaw PJ, Walls TJ, Newman PK, Cleland PG, Cartlidge NE. Hashimoto's encephalopathy: a steroid-responsive disorder associated with high anti-thyroid antibody titers-report of 5 cases. *Neurology.* 1991;41:228–233.

3. de Cerqueira AC, Bezerra JM, de Magalhaes GC, Rozenthal M, Nardi AE. Hashimoto's encephalopathy with clinical features similar to those of Creutzfeldt-Jakob disease. *Arq Neuropsiquiatr* 2008;66:903–905.

4. Matsunaga A, Ikawa M, Fujii A, et al. Hashimoto's encephalopathy as a treatable adult-onset cerebellar ataxia mimicking spinocerebellar degeneration. *Eur Neurol.* 2013;69:14–20.

5. Ishitobi M, Yoneda M, Ikawa M, et al. Hashimoto's encephalopathy with hippocampus involvement detected on continuous arterial spin labeling. *Psychiatry Clin Neurosci.* 2013;67:128–129.

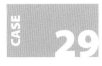

A Man with Urinary Incontinence and Trouble Walking

Linyan Tong, Kok Pin Ng, Yuxue Feng, Yu Li, Zongyi Xie, and Xiaofeng Li

29.1 Case History

A 71-year-old man was admitted for gradually difficult walking for 3 years along with memory impairment and urinary incontinence for 1 year. At first, this patient just complained of weakness while walking and dizziness. He was treated for arterial hypertension; however, no relief was obtained. He experienced more difficulties in walking and initiating steps. Besides these symptoms, his memory and thinking ability declined. His wife found that he responded slowly with personality change from a talkative and considerate gentleman to a silent man with apathy. The patient often felt urinary urgency, sometimes with incontinence. It was considered as symptoms of prostate hypertrophy. He was referred to a neurologist and MRI reported some lacunar infarctions and brain atrophy (retrospectively, lateral ventricles enlargement already existed). His Mini-Mental State Examination (MMSE) score was 18 points. Lumbar puncture (LP) was performed and cerebrospinal fluid (CSF) results were normal. The patient was diagnosed as having vascular dementia, hypertension and treated with neuroprotective agents and antihypertensives. After hospitalization, his symptoms were temporarily and partially relieved. His MMSE score was improved to 24 points when he was discharged.

Afterward, the patient still had symptoms as above. Two years later, the patient was referred to a neurosurgeon. Recognition and short-term memory had declined and head CT showed hydrocephalus with lacunar infarctions. LP was performed again. Intracranial pressure was 100 mm H_2O; however, a formal assessment of gait after the CSF tap was not performed.

Six years after the onset of symptoms the patient's symptoms further worsened. He could only slowly move on a smooth surface with the support of walking stick, although the muscle strength of his legs was normal. He lost the ability to communicate and could not attend social gatherings. He began to use diapers because of frequent urinary incontinence. A ventriculoperitoneal shunt was performed. One year after surgery the head CT showed hydrocephalus with no obvious change compared with last time. In the next 2 years of irregular follow-ups, the patient's condition was stable. His wife felt the patient appeared a little bit better after adjusting the pressure of the shunt. During the year before the last follow-up, the patient had small cerebral hemorrhages twice, in the pons and the left thalamus, respectively. At the last visit, the patient was conscious, could move in a wheel-chair and walk several steps with support, could answer his own name in a low voice and shake hands with visitors, wearing diapers, MMSE score was 4 points.

29.2 Discussion

Idiopathic normal pressure hydrocephalus (iNPH) was first described by Hakim and Adams in 1965, with a typical clinical triad of gait disturbance, cognitive impairment, and urinary incontinence in elderly patients, associated with enlargement of the cerebral ventricular system and good response to shunt surgery.[1] iNPH is an age-related disorder and its prevalence increases with age. In a community-based elderly population epidemiology study prevalence was about 1.4% in elderly adults. In a large elderly population in Sweden, the prevalence of probable iNPH was 0.2% in those aged 70–79 years and 5.9% in those aged 80 years and older. However, due to the subtle clinical onset and nonspecific nature of the clinical symptoms, the early diagnosis for iNPH is often challenging.

In this case, the patient was not diagnosed appropriately until 3 years later. Though the triad of gait disturbance, cognitive impairment, and urinary incontinence were present, each symptom was attributed to other diseases instead of iNPH. At first, dizziness was explained as the result of hypertension and the cognitive impairment was ignored and later interpreted as vascular dementia. Gait disturbance was misunderstood as fatigue and weakness of legs, even though the strength of the legs was confirmed to be normal. Urinary incontinence was noticed; however, it was explained as the result of prostate hypertrophy. Therefore understanding the clinical manifestation of iNPH is important.

29.2.1 Gait Disturbance

Gait disturbance is most likely the earliest and the most frequent symptom or sign that can be noticed. In the early course of the disease, the gait disturbance may be subtle and indistinguishable from careful senile gait. Patients may describe themselves as feeling dizzy or unstable as in this case. Later on, gait becomes evidently unstable and it may adopt a shuffling appearance similar to parkinsonian gait disorders. Patients then may complain of leg weakness, although formal neurologic assessment usually does not show motor deficits. iNPH gait is characterized by diminished gait velocity, mostly due to a diminished stride length, reduced step height, decreased foot-to-floor clearance, slow movement of the lower extremities, and a prominent disturbance of dynamic equilibrium, which was clearly distinguishable from the gait of patients with Parkinson's disease. The number of steps may be increased on turning. Findings include difficulty with movements; gait initiation failure; falling or festination; unstable multistep turns. The unique gait disturbance of iNPH with further progression of the disease are described as magnetic gait or as walking as if the feet were glued to the floor.[2]

29.2.2 Cognitive Impairment

Cognitive deficits are almost always present; however, they may also be subtle and even unrecognized in the early phase of the disease and may be detected only by neuropsychological examination. Patients with iNPH exhibit subcortical-type mental deficits that differ from that of Alzheimer's disease (AD). Common features include mental and motor slowing, apathy, emotional indifference, anosognosia, impaired memory and attention, decreased speed of information-processing and impaired executive function, including difficulty managing finances, taking medications properly, driving, and keeping track of appointments.[2]

29.2.3 Urinary Incontinence

Urgency and frequency are the most common urinary symptoms and may occur with or without incontinence. Urinary urgency without manifest incontinence is often observed in the early stage. Urodynamic testing has shown hyperreflexia and instability of the bladder detrusor muscle.

29.3 Quantitatively Evaluate Clinical Manifestations

The diagnosis of iNPH and appropriate selection of iNPH patients for shunt operation largely depend on accurate assessment of the change of clinical manifestation before and after the diagnostic tests (we will mention details later), it is therefore of great importance to quantitatively evaluate the clinical manifestation of iNPH.

29.3.1 Neuropsychological

Simple and easy screening tests such as the Mini-Mental State Examination (MMSE) or Montreal Cognitive Assessment (MoCA) are advised. As cognitive deficits in iNPH mainly consist of recall problems, adequate psychometric "frontal" tests such as Trail-Making Tests B and C, the Symbol Digit Memory Test, and the Stroop test are suggested. In the early stages, the cognitive profile is characterized mainly by impairments of attention, psychomotor speed, and memory, suggesting frontal involvement; patients with more advanced iNPH show overall cognitive deterioration.

29.3.2 Gait Disturbance

Quantitative gait assessment in iNPH is important due to the poor self-evaluation of the patients. The maximal increase in gait velocity can be observed 24–48 hours after the LP. This time point is also best to predict the response to shunting. The Timed Up and Go Test (TUG) is a standardized assessment in which a patient is observed and timed while arising from an arm chair, walking 3 m, turning around, walking back, and sitting down again. Dual-task walking (walking and backward counting) is another sensible method for gait evaluation.

29.3.3 Urinary Incontinence

The International Consultation on Incontinence Questionnaire – Short Form can be used.

29.4 Auxiliary Examinations

Auxiliary examinations can help diagnose iNPH early. Furthermore, due to irreversibility of the advanced stage and comorbidities of other degenerative diseases, some auxiliary examinations (diagnostic tests) have been investigated as to selecting the appropriate candidates for shunt surgery.

29.4.1 Brain Imaging

Computed tomography (CT) of the brain usually demonstrates symmetric widening of the lateral ventricles and the third ventricle. The ventriculomegaly may be quantified by assessment of the Evans index, which is the maximal frontal horn width divided by the transverse inner diameter of the skull at the same level (Figure 29.1). The fourth ventricle may or may not be dilated.

Magnetic resonance imaging (MRI) is informative in patients with suspected iNPH. The extent and severity of periventricular and deep white matter lesions can be better delineated. The sulcal flattening over the convexity can be evaluated much more easily with coronal imaging. The degree of dilatation of the perihippocampal fissures (PHF) may help differentiate iNPH from Alzheimer's disease, which has a relatively wider PHF.

29.4.2 Tap Test

Tap test, also known as the large-volume lumbar puncture (LP), is the most easily performed method. Transient improvement of gait disturbance after removal of 30–50 mL CSF via lumbar puncture indicates positive tap test. Several tap tests can be tried. However, negative tap test cannot exclude diagnosis of iNPH or positive response to shunt surgery. Unfortunately, in the case mentioned above, the patient has never been assessed with this method.

29.4.3 Continuous External Lumbar CSF Drainage

This method has been reported to have a high accuracy in predicting outcome after shunting. Daily 100–200 mL CSF is drained for a period of 3–5 days. The patient in this case was not evaluated with this method, either. If neither tap test nor continuous external lumbar CSF drainage showed any improvement, the patient could be avoided unnecessary operation.

29.5 How to Diagnose INPH?

iNPH is a clinical diagnosis that is based on medical history, neurologic examination, and brain imaging with CT or MRI. Both the international guideline[4] and the Japanese guidelines[5] of iNPH describe diagnostic criteria for iNPH. Briefly, patients with possible or probable iNPH present with one or more of the iNPH symptoms with insidious onset over 3 months or more, have an MRI or CT that shows ventriculomegaly, which cannot be explained by other diseases.[3] The Japanese guidelines will elevate diagnosis of possible iNPH to probable if diagnostic tests are positive or definitive if responsive to shunt surgery.

Concerning this case, the patient can be diagnosed as probable iNPH according to the international guideline. As this patient did not perform CSF removal test or lumbar drainage test and the shunt operation did not produce a good outcome, a diagnosis of possible iNPH can be made.

29.6 Differential Diagnosis

The most important differential diagnoses of iNPH of the elderly are subcortical vascular encephalopathy (SVE), Alzheimer's disease (AD), and Parkinson's disease (PD).

Symptoms of iNPH of the elderly and SVE may be very similar. Usually, subcortical dementia is more pronounced in advanced SVE, while the early appearance of gait disturbance and its dominance during the later course is supportive of iNPH though in some patients co-occurrence of iNPH and SVE had already been noted.

Compared with AD, attention and execution of iNPH patients are more impaired than memory and images may show narrower PHF. However, comorbidity with AD has been confirmed in several studies.

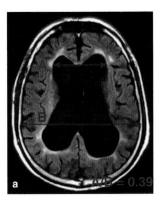

Figure 29.1 Evans Index (EI) = A/B, A: maximum diameter of frontal horn, B: maximum diameter of skull.

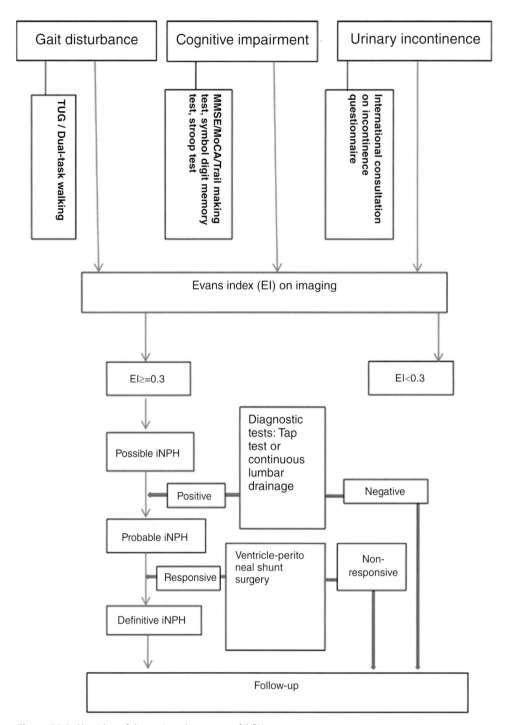

Figure 29.2 Algorithm of diagnosis and treatment of iNPH.

Gait disturbance may make iNPH misdiagnosed as PD. Careful examination of the tone of extremities may differentiate iNPH from PD.

29.7 Treatment

Until now, the underlying mechanism of iNPH is still unclear, it is generally accepted that the pathophysiological mechanisms involve reduced cerebral blood flow (CBF), a reduction in intracranial compliance, and a disturbance of CSF homeostasis. In the early stage, improvement of cerebral circulation has partly relieved some symptoms of this patient with increase in MMSE score from 18 to 24, which was assumed partly because of increase of periventricular blood flow. Until now, no drugs are effective in iNPH and specifically, no evidence supports the use of acetazolamide.[3] Shunt operation is the main effective treatment for iNPH, though this patient did not have good outcome of operation due to evolution into advanced stage and comorbidities with cerebrovascular diseases.

29.8 When to Initiate the Shunt Operation?

On the one hand, early treatment of iNPH may yield better postoperative outcomes. On the other hand, only one-third of patients enjoyed continued improvement by 3 years and complications occurred in 33% of patient. When is the appropriate time to initiate shunt operation? How to choose appropriate patients for shunt operation? However, the clinical presentation of iNPH by itself is usually not sufficient to recommend shunt surgery, as each of the primary iNPH symptoms has multiple potential etiologies and enlarged ventricles can be seen either with hydrocephalus or with brain atrophy. Therefore, it is necessary to predict the effects of shunt surgery before carrying out the operation. Predictive tests (the CSF tap test or continuous lumbar drainage) to determine the likelihood of shunt responsiveness are recommended. If multiple comorbidities or differential diagnoses make the diagnosis uncertain, referral to specialized centers that can perform ancillary tests can help to select patients with a high likelihood of responding to shunt surgery.

29.9 Longitudinal Follow-up after Shunt

Patients who have had shunt surgery should have periodic follow-up visits covering all three iNPH symptoms of gait impairment, incontinence, and dementia. Periodic brain imaging is recommended to look for signs of overdrainage, such as subdural effusion or hematoma, particularly in the first 6–12 months after shunt surgery until the patient's condition is stable. Symptoms of shunt malfunction or obstruction and disconnection of the shunt components should be explored.

29.10 Summary

Suspected iNPH patients should be given diagnostic CSF removal tests and those patients at a late stage should be selected very carefully. If there is secondary deterioration of the clinical symptoms after initial successful improvement after CSF shunting, shunt dysfunction should be ruled out aggressively (Figure 29.2).

References

1. Adams RD, Fisher CM, Hakim S, Ojemann RG, Sweet WH. Symptomatic occult hydrocephalus with "normal" cerebrospinal-fluid pressure. A treatable syndrome. *N Engl J Med.* 1965;273:117–126.

2. Krauss JK, von Stuckrad-Barre SF. Clinical aspects and biology of normal pressure hydrocephalus. *Handb Clin Neurol.* 2008;89:887–902.

3. Williams MA, Malm J. Diagnosis and treatment of idiopathic normal pressure hydrocephalus. *Continuum.* 2016;22:579–599.

4. Relkin N, Marmarou A, Klinge P, Bergsneider M, Black PM. Diagnosing idiopathic normal-pressure hydrocephalus. *Neurosurgery.* 2005;57:4–16.

5. Ishikawa M, Hashimoto M, Kuwana N, et al. Guidelines for management of idiopathic normal pressure hydrocephalus. *Neurol Med Chir.* 2008;48: 1–23.

Something Very Wrong Happened Very Fast

Mindy Halper, Calen Freeman, M. Uri Wolf, and Morris Freedman

30.1 Clinical History

Mr. C, a 75-year-old man, noticed difficulty remembering names and adding numbers after wakening while on vacation. Although these problems were quite subtle, his wife was puzzled because he seemed to have no difficulty the day before. One week later, he noted that "something was wrong" but could not describe the changes in detail. He felt that his balance was "not right" and experienced difficulty keeping track of his golf scores. Over the next few months, he developed word-finding problems and had difficulty expressing himself. He was very forgetful, had trouble problem solving, was distractible, and was unable to do simple calculations. Whereas he had previously been very reserved, he started talking with others in a more open way than he would normally have done. He continued to complain of balance problems and started to notice changes in his handwriting.

Mr. C was seen by his primary care physician who referred him to a geriatric psychiatrist. He was then referred to a neurologist. Six months after the onset of symptoms, he was seen in our Memory Disorders Clinic. By this time, he had significant difficulty communicating and was unable to take care of his finances. However, he continued to remain independent in basic activities of daily living. His wife experienced challenges in coping with the unexplained changes happening to her husband.

30.2 General History

Mr. C was born in Canada and had 16 years of education. He was married with children. He retired from his position as a high-level executive of a major corporation 10 years prior to presentation. He had a history of migraine-type headaches, hypertension, bladder cancer, skin cancer, and bilateral Dupuytren contractures. He also had a renal mass that was suspicious for a renal cell carcinoma. There was no family history of a neurodegenerative disorder.

30.3 Examination

Neurological examination performed 6 months after onset of symptoms was remarkable for bilateral grasp reflexes. He had agraphesthesia in both hands. There was mildly reduced arm swing on the right. Plantar responses were equivocal bilaterally. He displayed a full range of affect. He had significant word-finding difficulties and difficulty with simple mathematical calculations. Score on the Montreal Cognitive Assessment (MoCA) was 17/30.

30.4 Special Studies

Neuropsychology assessment was completed 3 months after onset of symptoms. This showed impairment in the following domains: auditory and visual working memory; mental tracking and processing speed; arithmetic ability (thought to be related mainly to working memory); and clock reading. Semantic fluency was more impaired than phonemic fluency. He had difficulty with word and memory retrieval.

Speech-language pathology assessment was completed 8 months after onset of symptoms. He was impaired in word finding, naming, reading, and writing with patterns of surface dyslexia and dysgraphia. Semantic knowledge was intact. There was no profile specific to any variant of primary progressive aphasia. Motor speech was intact, i.e. there was no evidence of dysarthria or apraxia of speech.

Single-photon emission computed tomography (SPECT) scan of the brain at 6 months after onset of symptoms showed mildly reduced perfusion in the high left parietal lobe and inferior right temporal lobe. Although magnetic resonance imaging (MRI) at 4 months was normal, repeat MRI at 8 months showed bilateral symmetrical cortical diffusion restriction and T2-fluid-attenuated inversion recovery (FLAIR) signal abnormality in the posterior aspect of both cerebral hemispheres involving the occipital and posterior temporoparietal lobes, as well as the frontal lobes. There was no involvement of the basal ganglia (Figure 30.1). These findings were highly suspicious for Creutzfeldt-Jakob disease (CJD).

Electroencephalogram (EEG) at 6 months was interpreted as normal. Repeat EEG at 8 months showed a slow background. However, no typical characteristics of CJD were seen.

(a) (b)

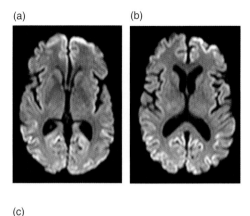

(c)

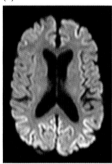

Figure 30.1(a–c) Bilateral symmetrical cortical diffusion restriction seen on DWI. This is most pronounced in the posterior region of both hemispheres but also involves the frontal lobes. There is no involvement of the basal ganglia.

Blood and cerebrospinal fluid (CSF) tests showed no evidence of infectious, autoimmune, or paraneoplastic disorders.

30.5 Diagnosis

Mr. C presented with an acute onset of a rapidly progressive dementia and had neuroimaging evidence suggestive of CJD. Other conditions including infection, autoimmune disorders, and paraneoplastic syndromes were excluded. Thus, a preliminary diagnosis of sporadic CJD was made.

30.6 Follow-Up

There was a progressive decline in all cognitive domains. By 15 months post onset, Mr. C was severely impaired cognitively, as well as functionally, and exhibited agitation and aggression. He was difficult to manage at home and was subsequently admitted to hospital on a geriatric unit for management. Although his agitation and aggression improved,

ambulation became problematic with the development of a spastic gait.

Furthermore, Mr. C developed increased deep tendon reflexes and a pill-rolling tremor in the right hand with marked increased tone in his upper extremities and increased axial tone. He had a broad-based apraxic gait. He ultimately developed a urinary tract infection with delirium and worsening confusion and agitation. He was transferred to a palliative care unit and died 18 months after onset. The disease process and symptoms were distressing to both Mr. C and his family who received ongoing support from the interprofessional team. This included linking to outside resources to address the psychosocial impact and stressors associated with his condition.

30.7 Autopsy

Histology and immunohistochemistry were consistent with CJD. The findings were not those found in histologically recognizable inherited forms of CJD.

30.8 Discussion

CJD is a rare and fatal rapidly progressive dementia. There are three major categories of CJD: hereditary, acquired (including variant), and sporadic, with the latter accounting for at least 85% of cases. Sporadic CJD (sCJD) progresses rapidly from often poorly defined prodromal symptoms to significant behavioral, cognitive, and motor abnormalities. Median time to death from onset is 5 months with 90% of patients dying within 1 year. Survival up to 72 months after onset of symptoms has been reported.[1] A conformational change in the prion protein ultimately leads to neuropathological findings of neuronal loss and vacuolization within cell bodies and dendrites that give a spongiform appearance to the cortex and deep nuclei. Immunocytochemical staining and western blot analysis demonstrate the presence of the pathogenic conformation of prion protein.

Mr. C presented with a slightly longer survival but an otherwise typical course of rapid progression involving cognitive, behavioral, and motor findings leading to death in 18 months. The acute onset of symptoms and lack of initial diagnostic investigations led to consideration of various diagnoses from a number of different specialists, an experience not uncommon in individuals with CJD or other rare

133

diseases. A diagnosis of stroke, vasculitis, Alzheimer's disease, primary progressive aphasia, and paraneoplastic syndrome were entertained. Repeating EEG and MRI after further disease progression were necessary to clarify diagnosis. Although the EEG did not show common findings of periodic sharp-wave complexes, repeat MRI showed cortical ribboning consistent with sCJD. Exclusion of other diagnoses through serum and CSF investigations led to the diagnosis of sCJD, which was confirmed at autopsy.

Evidence suggests that there is often a delay in the diagnosis of sCJD. Significant heterogeneity of initial presentation, presence of psychiatric symptoms, and a range of neurological symptoms pose a challenge with triaging the assessment and care of individuals with suspected sCJD.[2] Misdiagnosis may also be due in part to the insensitivity of sCJD criteria to early symptoms of the disease, the rarity of the condition, heterogeneity of symptoms, and a symptom profile that overlaps with other neurodegenerative conditions.[3] These challenges, together with the need for prompt and accurate diagnosis, have led to the suggestion that CJD be considered in any rapidly progressive dementia whenever a differential diagnosis includes neurodegenerative, autoimmune, infectious, or toxic/metabolic conditions.[2]

Patients with rare diseases often face considerable obstacles in accessing and navigating the healthcare system. The delays in diagnosis, scarcity of skilled and experienced healthcare providers, and lack of peer and psychosocial supports experienced by patients and family are common themes in the literature on CJD and other rare disorders.

To ease diagnosis, healthcare professionals are trained to recognize a set list of symptoms. However, Mr. C's symptoms did not fit into any neat textbook diagnostic boxes. With rare diseases, one specialty or clinician is usually insufficient to diagnose and manage the condition. Patients often need to see a variety of specialists for different aspects of their care. Within months of referral to our center, Mr. C had been seen by numerous clinicians from various disciplines. Involvement of an occupational therapist, registered nurse, social worker, psychologist, psychiatrist, neurologist, speech-language pathologist, radiologist, and disease-specific associations were all important aspects of care. Evidence suggests that a coordinated, comprehensive, and multidisciplinary approach to assessment, diagnosis, and care may lead to improved symptoms and quality of life for

individuals and families, even with fatal conditions. Despite the rapid progression and fatal outcome, the support received by Mr. C and his family from the various healthcare team members throughout the course of his illness had significant positive impact on their experience. However, merely seeing individual clinicians is rarely sufficient to support effective assessment and care for patients. The care should be coordinated and address the psychosocial needs of patients and families. Our ability to provide efficient and effective assessment and care was contingent on the coordination of all services. The continued involvement of nursing staff ensured that the burden of coordinating care did not fall entirely to the patient's family. In addition to supporting the assessment process, team members were able to provide counseling, education, and assistance in navigating other health services.

Patient perceptions that healthcare professionals have failed to meet their expectations is cited as the primary source of difficulties when confronted with a rare disease.[4] Expectations reflect the need to feel informed, supported, and listened to, rather than only to obtain information about disease-specific processes. Regardless of the availability of medical information or treatment options, the ability of healthcare professionals to provide this ongoing support is a key factor associated with a positive disease experience.[4] A challenge in this case was the capacity of the individual clinicians in working with individuals with CJD. Given the rarity of the condition, few had experience working with individuals with CJD. Clinicians drew on their expertise in working with individuals with other rare or rapidly progressive illnesses and acquired additional knowledge through working closely with peers and disease-specific organizations. Efforts and advice regarding strategies to improve daily life were frequent topics of conversation with the patient and his family and have demonstrated ability to improve the experience of individuals and families.[4] For example, initiating a transparent discussion regarding safe driving early allowed the patient to be informed about potential risks, maintain independence, and participate in discussions about mitigating risk, ultimately resulting in driving cessation.

There is a body of evidence suggesting that a rare disease can incite feelings of isolation, invisibility, and powerlessness.[3] Themes of discussion with the patient and family included fear, anxiety, and distress. They were eager to know everything they could about the condition, prognosis, expected course of illness, and available support services. They wanted to plan their lives and future. Their psychosocial and emotional distress were compounded by limited information and access to peer support services. Aside from the expected distress from dealing with an unknown diagnosis and prognosis, the patient and family experienced challenges in dealing with practical issues such as insurance and accommodation of travel plans.

Connecting with peers can have a significant impact on these experiences. Learning about potential treatments, community resources, research, and even just hearing about the experiences of others can help break the isolation that individuals with rare conditions often report. In the absence of organized peer support organizations, many individuals turn to online sources of information. Online sources can provide high-quality evidence-based information. On the other hand, they can provide inaccurate and, at times, dangerous information. A quick internet search of CJD reveals sites dedicated to the research and treatment of prion diseases. This also reveals sites devoted to sharing fanatical stories about outbreaks of mad cow disease, isolation, and cannibalism. For patients like Mr. C, the line between good and bad can be blurred. Technology can empower them and break their isolation. However, it does not replace the information and support required from trained healthcare professionals. Mr. C's family relied on the ongoing availability of support from nursing, medicine, and social work. This afforded them the opportunity to access high-quality evidence-based information about disease processes, symptom control, and community supports.

Trying to find a diagnosis for a rare condition can be a long and frustrating experience. Both Mr. C and his family communicated significant distress, not only from the burden of the symptoms but as a direct result of the frustration and fear experienced in being diagnosed with sCJD. It helps to work with the individual and family to understand their experiences and observations and to explain to them symptoms and procedures. Despite being considered a fatal condition, the prompt and precise diagnosis of CJD can have significant impact on patient outcomes and experience. It allows individuals and families to anticipate care needs, identify goals for care, enlist supports and resources, and have open discussions regarding powers of attorney and end-of-life care planning. Collaboration among team members and with partner organizations allowed our team to share collective knowledge and build capacity and expertise in the holistic care of an individual with CJD.

30.9 Take-Home Message

The precise in vivo and pathological diagnosis of rare cause of dementias has significant impact on patient outcomes.

Acknowledgments

M. Freedman receives support from the Saul A. Silverman Family Foundation as a Canada International Scientific Exchange Program and Morris Kerzner Memorial Fund.

References

1. Puoti G, Bizzi A, Forloni G, et al. Sporadic human prion disease: molecular insights and diagnosis. *Lancet Neurol.* 2012;11:618–628.

2. Paterson RW, Torres-Chae CC, Kuo AL, et al. Differential diagnosis of Jakob-Creutzfeldt disease. *Arch Neurol.* 2012;69 (12):1578–1582.

3. Rabinovici GD, Wang PN, Levin J, et al. First symptom in sporadic Creutzfeldt–Jakob disease. *Neurology.* 2006;66(2):286–287.

4. Huyard C. What, if anything, is specific about having a rare disorder? Patients' judgements on being ill and being rare. *Health Expect.* 2009;12 (4):361–370.

Siblings with a Fatal Cause of Rapidly Progressive Dementia

Tharick A. Pascoal, Mira Chamoun, Sara Mohades, Monica Shin,
Liyong Wu, Serge Gauthier, and Pedro Rosa-Neto

31.1 Case Histories

A 62-year-old male (Patient 1) was admitted to the Capital Medical University Hospital, in Beijing, China, because of a 3-month history of progressive cognitive impairment and abnormal behaviors including performing motor gestures and talking to himself incoherently. During the first evaluation, it was reported that the patient had insomnia as an early clinical manifestation accompanied by intense dreams and sleep talking. During the 14 days of hospitalization, the patient showed intractable insomnia, progressive cognitive deterioration, mental confusion, visual and auditory hallucinations, and paranoia. Twelve months after the onset of the symptoms, the patient returned to the hospital awake but unresponsive and died due to breathing difficulties.

The patient's younger sister, a 60-year-old woman (Patient 2) with no education, was assessed after the first hospitalization of her brother. She reported a 5-month history of cognitive and mental symptoms accompanied by sleep disturbance for 2 months. The patient's first symptoms included panic attacks, fatigue during daytime, apathy, disinterests in work, and lack of engagement in conversation with friends and family members. Two months later, the patient showed difficulties in falling asleep at night, limb movements during sleep, diurnal somnolence, and oneiric behaviors. In the subsequent months, despite the use of many different sleep inductors, her insomnia continued to worsen, and her symptoms evolved to severe hallucinations, impaired memory, incoherent speech, unsteady gaits, changes in voice, and increased sweating. She was never hospitalized and passed away at home with a symptom described as a severe dyspnea.

31.2 Medical History

Both siblings had no relevant previous medical history.

31.3 Family History

The patients' mother and an older brother had similar symptoms with rapidly progressive dementia and death.

31.4 First Clinical Assessment

(Patient 1): A heart rate of 105 beats/min, BP of 160/100 mmHg, cranial nerves normal, muscle strength and tension normal, reflexes normal and symmetric, Babinski negative, and scored 4 points in Mini–Mental State Examination (MMSE). Additionally, the patient showed anisocoria with impaired direct and consensual pupillary light reflexes of the left eye.

(Patient 2): A heart rate of 108 beats/min, BP of 160/90 mmHg, normal cranial nerves, normal muscle strength and tone, reflexes normal and symmetric, Babinski negative, scored 4 points in the MMSE and 3 points in the clinical dementia rating scale.

31.5 Additional Assessments

The patients underwent a lumbar puncture, an electroencephalogram, a polysomnography (PSG), neuroimaging, and genetic assessments.

31.5.1 Cerebrospinal Fluid

(Patient 1): A cerebrospinal fluid pressure of 150 mm H_2O (normal value, 100–180), sugar of 80 mg/dL (normal value, 45–80), chloride of 109 mmol/L (normal value, 118–128), protein of 16 mg/dL (normal, 15–45), white blood cells of 0 mm^3 (normal, 0), and 14-3-3 protein negative.

(Patient 2): A cerebrospinal fluid pressure of 150 mm H_2O, sugar of 74 mg/dL, chloride of 107 mmol/L, protein of 26 mg/dL, white blood cells of 0 mm^3, and 14-3-3 protein negative.

31.5.2 Electroencephalogram

(Patient 1): The basic rhythm was 10 c/s with amplitude slow waves at 3–7 Hz.

(Patient 2): The basic rhythm was 9 c/s with amplitude slow waves at 5–7 Hz.

31.5.3 Polysomnography

(Patient 1): The polysomnography showed reduced sleep efficiency, prolonged sleep latency, normal awakening, abnormal sleep architecture, reduced stage I, reduced proportion of stage II, increased proportion of deep sleep, reduction of the rapid sleep eye movement (REM) period, obstructive sleep apnea events (minimum oxygen saturation 83%), and involuntary lower limb movements mainly occurring in stage II (Figure 31.1).

(Patient 2): The polysomnography showed reduced sleep efficiency, normal sleep latency, increased awakening, disordered sleep structure, poor sleep cycle progression, slightly increased proportion of stage I, increased proportion of deep sleep, and reduction of the REM period. After falling asleep, the patient had throat sounds and a large number of involuntary upper and lower limb movements mainly occurring in stage II, as well as mild sleep apnea (minimum blood oxygen saturation of 89%) (Figure 31.1).

31.5.4 Neuroimaging

(Patient 1): The magnetic resonance image (MRI) was normal. However, the single-photon emission computed tomography (SPECT) demonstrated a decline in perfusion in the thalamus bilaterally, basal ganglia, and the medial temporal cortex.

(Patient 2): The MRI was normal. However, the [18F]fluorodeoxyglucose positron emission tomography (PET) indicated decreased uptake in the left thalamus and inferior parietal lobe bilaterally.

31.5.5 Genetic Assessment

Gene sequencing of DNA extracted from the peripheral blood leukocytes revealed that both patients had a D178N mutation with methionine/methionine homozygosity at the polymorphic codon 129 of the PRNP gene. Seven family members of the patients were

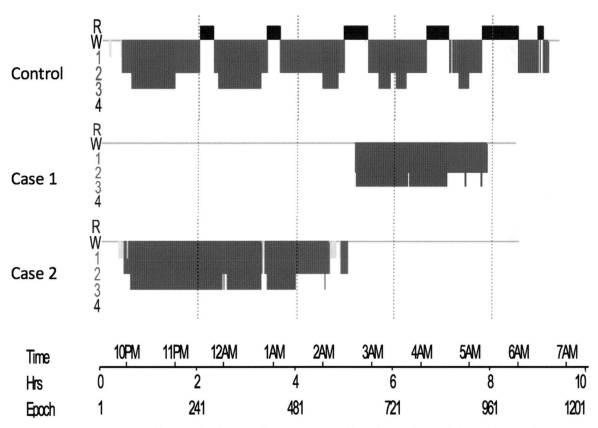

Figure 31.1 Hypnogram of a healthy control and the two FFI patients presented here showing decreased sleep efficiency and disruption of the normal cyclic sleep organization (horizontal axis represents sleep hours). FFI: fatal familial insomnia, W: wake, R: REM, N1–3: non-REM sleep stages.

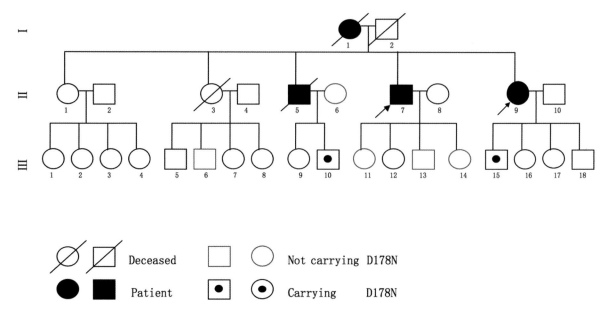

Deceased   Not carrying D178N

Patient   Carrying   D178N

Figure 31.2 The pedigrees of the seven family members that were screened for the PRNP gene mutation.

screened for PRNP gene mutation. The other family members were not screened due to lack of consent or prior death. Results of the screened family members are demonstrated in Figure 31.2.

31.6 Diagnosis

Both patients presented here suffered from fatal familial insomnia (FFI). FFI is a rare autosomal dominant disease characterized by predominant thalamic degeneration. Patients suffering from FFI have intractable sleep disturbance, loss of coordination, and decline of mental functions. Death follows within months to a few years after the appearance of initial symptoms.

31.7 Discussion

These two cases demonstrate an extremely rare cause of rapidly progressive dementia. Fatal familial insomnia (FFI) is an autosomal dominant prion disease first described in 1986 and with only about 30 families having been described in the literature so far.

FFI affects men and women equally, with an age of onset around 50 years and death usually within 12–18 months. FFI is associated with a D178N mutation in the PRNP gene, which is reported in nearly all families with the disease. This mutation also occurs in familial Creutzfeldt-Jakob disease (fCJD). Evidence

suggests that patients with this mutation who are homozygous for methionine at codon 129 develop FFI syndrome, whereas individuals homozygous for valine develop fCJD. Interestingly, studies have reported considerable clinical and pathological overlaps between patients with the different types of D178N mutations, suggesting a continuous spectrum of the aforementioned prion diseases.

The predominant thalamic neuronal degeneration with deposition of the pathogenic prion protein (PrPSc) is the most prominent pathological feature of FFI affecting mainly the medio-dorsal and anterio-ventral nucleus. In addition, moderate atrophy of the cortex and basal ganglia have been reported in FFI patients. The thalamus is a brain region involved in the control of the sleep-wake cycle and in the "communication" between different brain regions. Therefore, the neuronal degeneration of the thalamus is postulated the main mechanism that FFI leads to its symptoms. However, it is well established that other mechanisms are not yet fully understood, including non-thalamic brain regions' role in this process. One may speculate that the hypothalamic and cortical hypometabolism reported here in these two cases further support the notion that the disrupted sleep arousal cycle in FFI may occur in part due to certain degree of impairment in the basal ganglia to cortex circuits.

The main clinical manifestations of FFI are intractable insomnia and sleep-wake cycle disruption. However, cognitive and behavioral disorders manifested as rapidly progressive dementia are often among the first symptoms. Other common symptoms include hallucinations, dreaminess, reduced sleep time, panic attacks, phobias, and weight loss. Symptoms related to autonomic dysfunctions are also common such as hypertension, hyperhidrosis, shortness of breath, and tachycardia. Additionally, some patients may suffer from ataxia, dysarthria, dysphagia, and pyramidal tract injury. PSG abnormalities are often present showing reduced sleep time, reduced REM sleep, and abnormal stage shifts. In some cases, FFI is characterized by the lack of muscle atonia in the REM sleep, a jerky activity of the limb muscle, and irregular breathing.

Several characteristics supported the diagnostic of FFI in the two cases presented here. They had the combination of rapidly progressive dementia, autonomic symptoms (hyperhidrosis, elevated blood pressure, and tachycardia), and severe insomnia that did not improve with the use of sleep inducers. The two patients had not only refractory insomnia but also laryngeal and involuntary movements during sleep, which are also reported in patients with FFI. It is noteworthy that we have shown for the first time here that the laryngeal and involuntary movements occurred in the non-REM stage II. Additionally, these cases had a clear family history with four patients in two generations affected, which is consistent with an autosomal dominant inheritance disorder. PSG examination revealed that the overall sleep time was shortened with disruptions of the normal cyclic sleep organization, the sleep spindle was significantly reduced, the slow waves during sleep were significantly reduced, and the REM sleep was reduced. The hypometabolism in the thalamus corroborated the clinical symptoms and, in the end, the genetic test confirmed the diagnosis of FFI in the family.

An important differential diagnosis in these cases is fCJD, which is another hereditary fatal prion disease. Although fCJD can also be characterized by rapidly progressive dementia and psychotic behaviors such as those presented by the two patients here, both patients had no myoclonic jerks and seizures that are commonly found in fCJD. Other characteristics that also helped to rule out fCJD were the lack of periodic discharges in the electroencephalogram and absence of the lace sign in brain MRI (DWI sequence), both typically found in fCJD. In the end, the genetic test suggested the diagnosis of FFI rather than fCJD in these individuals.

To date, there is no effective treatment to slow the progression of FFI. The main goals of the current treatments are to ease symptoms and bring comfort to the patients and their families. Although some treatments have shown delay in FFI progression in animal models, these results did not stand in the subsequent human studies. However, the current development of promising therapies such as immunotherapies in its different forms brings hope for patients with FFI in a near future.

One may conclude that for patients with rapidly progressive dementia, intractable sleep disorder, and compatible family history, the possibility of FFI should be considered. Characteristic sleep polygraph signs and thalamic hypometabolism are helpful, but only PRNP gene sequence analysis can confirm the diagnosis.

Further Reading

Lugaresi E, Medori R, Montagna P, et al. Fatal familial insomnia and dysautonomia with selective degeneration of thalamic nuclei. *N Engl J Med.* 1986;315 (16):997–1003.

Manetto V, Medori R, Cortelli P, et al. Fatal familial insomnia: clinical and pathologic study of five new cases. *Neurology.* 1992;42: 312–319.

Medori R, Tritschler HJ, LeBlanc A, et al. Fatal familial insomnia, a prion disease with a mutation at codon 178 of the prion protein gene. *N Engl J Med.* 1992;326:444–449.

Montagna P. Fatal familial insomnia: a model disease in sleep physiopathology. *Sleep Med Rev.* 2005;9:339–353.

Montagna P, Gambetti P, Cortelli P, Lugaresi E. Familial and sporadic fatal insomnia. *Lancet Neurol.* 2003;2:167–176.

Left or Right: Which Way to Go?

André Aguiar Souza Furtado de Toledo, Karoline Carvalho Carmona,
Leonardo Cruz de Souza, and Paulo Caramelli

32.1 Case History

A 73-year-old Brazilian, right-handed man, retired business manager, began having progressively cognitive and behavioral disorders for the past 5 years. His family noticed some behavioral changes, as he presented with great irritability, usage of bad language, profound inhibition, apathy, and unprecedented religious interests (hyper-religiosity). He had no history of hallucinations. During the consultation, the patient recurrently said in a delirious speech that he was a "disgrace," that he was disturbing his wife and family, and it would be a relief if he died. His conversation was predominantly melancholic and mostly about self-centered themes.

He also had difficulties with his memory. According to him, his "memory did not exist." He insidiously started to have problems in episodic memory. He noted he was having difficulty in retaining information from newspapers and TV shows, but still could remember numerical information and important meetings. He also started to have language problems, such as incapacity in understanding written material or comprehending complex speeches (e.g., concatenated ideas). Apparently his autonomy for daily life activities, like financial tasks and driving, remained preserved, although he decided to leave his job due to his cognitive problems. He had no history of traumatic brain injury, seizures, stroke, or alcoholism. He has a history of rheumatoid arthritis and current medications included nonsteroidal anti-inflammatory drugs and methotrexate. There was no family history of dementia.

On examination, the patient was alert and fully oriented. Cranial nerves were intact. On motor exam, his tone and power were normal, although he had increased reflexes globally. Gait, coordination, and sensory examination were normal, and there were no signs of parkinsonism. On cognitive testing, his performance in the Mini-Mental State Examination (MMSE) was 27/30 as he missed the three words on delayed recall. He did quite well in the Brief Cognitive Battery (BCB), presenting some difficulty naming simple figures such as key and turtle.[1] The clock-drawing test was normal. When asked to write irregular words, the patient miswrote less than a half of them (clinical profile compatible with surface dysgraphia). The physical examination was otherwise normal.

Screening laboratory tests for reversible causes of dementia were ordered and all results were within normal ranges, including blood count, comprehensive metabolic panel, thyroid-stimulating hormone, vitamin B12, and venereal disease research laboratory. A magnetic resonance imaging (MRI) was performed and revealed moderate atrophy of the right anterior temporal lobe. A new MRI (2 years later) demonstrated increase of the right anterior temporal atrophy and also atrophy involving the anterior parts of the left temporal lobe, although less severe (Figures 32.1 and 32.2). Single-photon emission computed tomography (SPECT) displayed focal hypoperfusion of the right temporal lobe.

Based on the overall clinical, neuropsychological, and neuroimaging data a probable diagnosis of frontotemporal dementia (right temporal variant) was made.

32.2 Discussion

Frontotemporal dementia (FTD) constitutes a group of neurodegenerative diseases that are clinically, pathologically, and genetically heterogeneous. It is known as a predominant early-onset dementia and is considered one of the most common causes of dementia in adults younger than 60 years of age, with the onset of symptoms typically occurring in the sixth decade of life. While the expression FTD refers to the clinical syndrome, frontotemporal lobar degeneration (FTLD) is related to the anatomical concept of selective neuronal degeneration in frontal and temporal lobes that is observed in most of the patients with FTD.[2,3]

The three major clinical presentations include the frontal or behavioral variant (bvFTD), the temporal variant (tvFTD; also known as semantic dementia, SD), and the progressive nonfluent aphasia (PNFA; also known as primary progressive aphasia nonfluent/

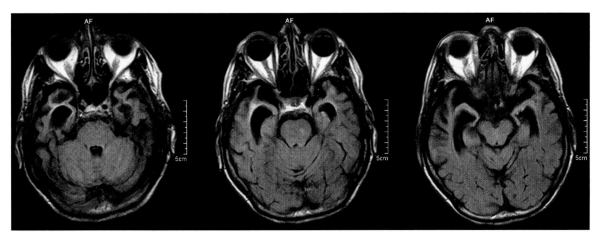

Figure 32.1 MRI (FLAIR sequence; axial slices) showing the temporal lobes at the level of the optic nerves. Note the atrophy of the anterior temporal lobes, most prominently in the right side (upper left side of the images).

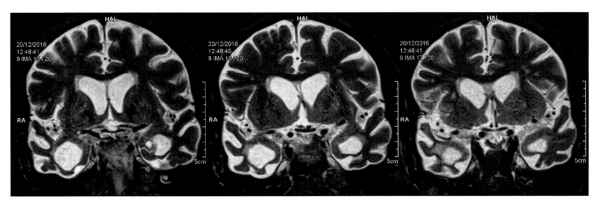

Figure 32.2 MRI (T2 sequence; coronal slices). Note the atrophy of the anterior temporal lobes, most prominently in the right side (lower left side of the images).

agrammatic type, nfPPA).[4] These clinical syndromes differ from each other by different atrophy patterns, which explain the degrees of personality change, executive dysfunction, and language impairment.

Patients diagnosed with bvFTD usually exhibit exuberant behavioral changes, like disinhibition, apathy, loss of empathy, ritualistic or stereotyped behaviors, hyperorality and changes in eating preferences. Moreover, these patients may show deficits in social cognition and executive functions. Neuroimaging studies typically indicates atrophy predominantly frontal-insular rather than temporal.[2] The bvFTD is by itself a heterogeneous disorder. A study conducted by Whitwell and colleagues with sixty-six subjects with clinical diagnosis of bvFTD

showed that patients within this clinical syndrome could be divided into four different subtypes on an anatomical basis – two of which are defined by important frontal atrophy and the other two by predominant temporal lobe atrophy. Moreover, the temporal prominent subtype showed different patterns of gray matter loss, since one was restricted to the inferior and medial lobes, especially in the right temporal lobe, named "temporal-dominant" subtype. Patients with this subtype performed worse on tests of naming and memory than the other three subtypes, as well as showed a high proportion of changes in appetite and eating behavior, without apathy as a common feature. These results confirmed that a right dominant temporal atrophy can occur in the context of bvFTD and not just in semantic dementia.[5]

Whereas in bvFTD, asymmetrical distribution of atrophy across the hemispheres is less frequent, in SD there is significant lateralization of atrophy, with the distribution of degeneration across hemispheres being highly asymmetrical, primarily in the early stages of the disease. Moreover, SD is associated with asymmetrical atrophy of the anterior temporal lobes, frequently greater on the left. Classic descriptions of SD used to emphasize the cognitive features of the disease, but recent studies found that behavioral symptoms are also common in this variant, simulating changes typically found in bvFTD.

In this context, a (new) variant has been described by an increasing number of case reports presenting patients with either progressive loss of self-identification and knowledge or prominent changes in behavior. However, there are still fewer case reports describing this clinical-genetic-pathological entity, named here as right temporal variant frontotemporal dementia (RtvFTD). The literature usually addresses the RtvFTD by three main perceptions: (1) an atypical form of bvFTD, as it exhibits an asymmetrical right temporal lobe atrophy (the temporal-dominant subtype described previously); (2) a subtype of the SD syndrome with a major involvement of the right temporal lobe and with more exuberant behavioral manifestation; and (3) a new anatomical variant of FTD, with some sort of clinical-pathological homogeneity.[6] As can be seen, the shortage of knowledge about RtvFTD makes it a still undefined entity, a disorder within a clinical-genetic-pathological gradient between bvFTD and SD (Figure 32.3).

It is known that patients with marked degeneration of the left (dominant) hemisphere commonly lose verbal semantic knowledge, characterized by word-finding difficulties and impaired comprehension, as well as stereotypical behaviors and changes in eating pattern. Conversely, right-sided atrophy patients exhibit inappropriate behaviors, including alterations in affect and in social conduct, with a typical lack of insight, aside from episodic memory deficits, difficulties in face recognition (prosopagnosia), and topographic disorientation. A study carried out by Josephs and colleagues characterized two phenotypes of the RtvFTD – bvFTD phenotype and SD phenotype –, with significant differences identified between both groups. The first was defined by personality changes, inappropriate behaviors and positive family history, in addition to poor performance on behavioral tests and better performance on naming tests. The second was defined by word-finding and oral comprehension difficulties, prosopagnosia and topographagnosia, as well as an absence of family history, better performance on behavioral tests and poor performance on naming tests.[6]

The patient described in this chapter had early decline in episodic memory. Although memory complaints are classically related to Alzheimer's disease

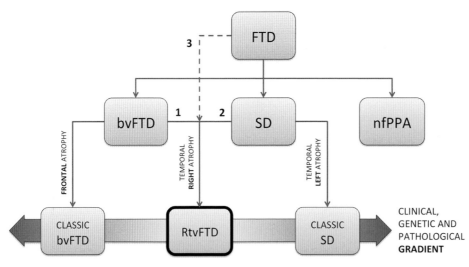

Figure 32.3 Clinical, genetic, and pathological model of right temporal variant frontotemporal dementia (RtvFTD). FTD: frontotemporal dementia. bvFTD: behavioral variant FTD. SD: semantic dementia. nfPPA: primary progressive aphasia nonfluent type.

(AD), recent studies describe different memory impairment patterns in the FTD variants.[7] The involvement of the anterior hippocampal region observed in SD corroborates the finding of markedly autobiographical memory loss rather than remote memory deficits that are usually found in AD.[7] The patient also presented with evident behavioral changes, like irritability, hyper-religiosity and apathy, as reported by his family. Changes in personality are a common early manifestation of RtvFTD.[6,8] Moreover, behavioral changes are more frequent in RtvFTD than in classic SD, mainly social behavioral changes and loss of insight.[4,6] Additionally, in this case, manifestations of language deficits described as word-finding and oral comprehension difficulties for complex material were reported, in association with naming difficulties and dysgraphia. The semantic processing of words and objects (naming, word comprehension and object recognition) is associated with the left anterior temporal lobe, while the right anterior temporal lobe is being increasingly related to empathy and emotional processing, multimodal semantic knowledge for faces and objects, eating behaviors, and nonverbal aspects of speech.[9]

A study carried by Thompson and colleagues managed to characterize the symptomatology in a series of forty-seven patients diagnosed with SD in order to investigate if the asymmetrical predominance of atrophy could produce distinct behavioral or cognitive profiles.[4] They found that the two groups of patients, named left predominant (L > R) and right predominant (R > L) variants showed significant differences in symptoms and performance in neuropsychological tests. The L > R patients generally had a greater deficit in naming tasks, depression as the major behavioral symptom, and hyperorality with a preference for sweet foods. In the other hand, the R > L group showed a relatively high number of subjects with changes in social behavior as the commonest behavioral symptom, with encompassed rude and tactless comments, as well as lack of insight and irritability. Considering the most prominent symptoms at presentation, the two groups showed interesting differences. In the R > L group, the main complaint was prosopagnosia (in more than 90% subjects), in addition to bizarre changes in affect and social awkwardness. In the L > R group, word-finding difficulties and impaired comprehension are the main clinical features, together with depression, stereotyped behaviors and changes in eating pattern.

R > L patients also exhibited lack of empathy and self-centeredness, which can be observed in the presented case.

Most FTD cases are sporadic, but approximately 15% of cases are related to an autosomal dominant genetic mutation. The three main subtypes of FTD are based on the type of inclusions found in the brain: tau, TDP-43 (transactive response DNA-binding protein 43), and FUS (RNA-binding protein fused in sarcoma). The most studied genes associated with FTD are MAPT (microtubule-associated protein tau), GRN (progranulin gene), and C9ORF72. In the study by Josephs and colleagues[6] cited previously, all subjects with the bvFTD phenotype had tau abnormalities, mostly related to mutations in the MAPT gene, while all the SD phenotype subjects had a pathology related to TDP-43. In the same way, a study carried out by Miller and colleagues evaluated 20 cases of RtvFTD and found that patients with more prominent behavioral symptoms had a tau protein mutation, while patients with significant language impairment had abnormalities in TDP-43. Finally, in the study conducted by Whitwell and colleagues, subjects with the temporal-dominant subtype of bvFTD had a positive family history for the disorder and a high prevalence of genetically confirmed mutations in MAPT.[2,5,6] Therefore, we can conclude that more than one mutation could be associated with the right temporal lobe atrophy of RtvFTD. Indeed, it should be emphasized that there is limited correlation between clinical phenotype and the histopathological type of FTD.

Neuroimaging studies are an important tool to evaluate patients with cognitive, behavioral or language symptoms in order to understand the pathological process of FTD. Patients with FTD classically present frontal and temporal lobe atrophy in structural studies, as in MRI of the brain, or hypometabolism in functional studies, as in positron-emission tomography (PET).[10] However, more detailed studies revealed the wide variety of atrophy patterns across patients, exhibiting variable frontal or temporal predominance, diverse levels of asymmetry, as well as the involvement of other cortical and subcortical areas.[10] PET with [^{18}F] fluorodeoxyglucose (FDG-PET) and SPECT are the most applied methods to investigate different patterns of cerebral glucose metabolism or cerebral perfusion. These patterns of hypometabolism/hypoperfusion estimate neuronal dysfunction and tend to have a reasonable correlation with patterns of atrophy.[10] MRI obtained from the patient shows a predominant atrophy of the right anterior temporal lobe, which illustrates the usual changes found in the RtvFTD. Likewise, SPECT of the patient reveals a mild hypoperfusion of the right temporal lobe, supporting the structural findings.

32.3 Take-Home Message

Imaging phenotype provides important insights regarding clinical diagnosis.

References

1. Nitrini R, Caramelli P, Herrera Junior E, et al. Performance of illiterate and literate nondemented elderly subjects in two tests of long-term memory. *J Int Neuropsychol Soc.* 2004;10:634–638.

2. Miller BL, Dickerson BC, Lucente DE, Larvie M, Frosch MP. Case 9-2015: a 31-year-old man with personality changes and progressive neurologic decline. Case records of the Massachusetts General Hospital. *N Engl J Med.* 2015;372:1151–1162.

3. Rohrer JD, Lashley T, Schott JM, et al. Clinical and neuroanatomical signatures of tissue pathology in frontotemporal lobar degeneration. *Brain.* 2011;134:2565–2581.

4. Thompson SA, Patterson K, Hodges JR. Left/right asymmetry of atrophy in semantic dementia: behavioral-cognitive implications. *Neurology.* 2003;61:1196–1203.

5. Whitwell JL, Przybelski SA, Weigand SD, et al. Distinct anatomical subtypes of the behavioural variant of frontotemporal dementia: a cluster analysis study. *Brain.* 2009;132:2932–2946.

6. Josephs KA, Whitwell JL, Knopman DS, et al. Two distinct subtypes of right temporal variant frontotemporal dementia. *Neurology.* 2009;73:1443–1450.

7. Hornberger M, Piguet O. Episodic memory in frontotemporal dementia: a critical review. *Brain.* 2012;135:678–692.

8. Seeley WW, Bauer AM, Miller BL, et al. The natural history of temporal variant frontotemporal dementia. *Neurology.* 2005;64:1384–1390.

9. Henry ML, Wilson SM, Ogar JM, et al. Neuropsychological, behavioral, and anatomical evolution in right temporal variant frontotemporal dementia: a longitudinal and post-mortem single case analysis. *Neurocase.* 2014;20:100–109.

10. Gordon E, Rohrer JD, Fox NC. Advances in neuroimaging in frontotemporal dementia. *J Neurochem.* 2016;138(Suppl. 1):193–210.

Young Woman with Problems Concentrating

Renaud David, Isabelle Gomez-Luporsi, Cindy Giaume, Elsa Leone, Aurélie Mouton, and Philippe Robert

33.1 Clinical History – Main Complaint

Ms. L is having a regular ongoing follow-up with a psychiatrist in private practice for a history of bipolar disorder (BP). She reported a first major depressive episode at the age of 17 as well as one manic episode several years later. She had a last depressive episode 10 years ago and is currently stabilized under antipsychotic medication. Before being prescribed antipsychotics, she was under sodium valproate medication. She also reported a suicide attempt at the age of 11. In addition to her BP, she reported a dysthyroidia treated with L-thyroxine.

Current medications: aripiprazole (Abilify®), L-thyroxine, cyproterone acetate (androcur®), biperidene chlorhydrate (akineton®).

Her main complaints, motivating the initial consultation, are memory disturbances for recent facts associated to attention and concentration disturbances, as well as phonemic and semantic paraphasia. Due to the reported disturbances, she should note everything she does, and, according to her children, constantly repeats the same things. All these symptoms started 2 years ago.

33.2 General History

Mrs. L (aged 55 at the first consultation) is married and has two children; she is currently working as a sculptor.

33.3 Family History

One grandmother had a probable Alzheimer's disease at the age of 60.

33.4 Examination

She appeared very anxious during the first consultation at both the testing and interview with a noticeable slowdown in thoughts, especially when initiating new tasks during the neurocognitive assessment, which showed the following results:

Mini Mental State Exam (MMSE): 30/30

Free and Cued Selective Reminding Test (Grober and Buschke): total score 48/48, immediate free recall 31/48, delayed free recall 16/16

Frontal Assessment Battery: 17/18 (normal performances)

Rey figure: memory score 15/36 (p < 10), 113 s (pathological performances)

Trail Making Test A: 30s (p50), Trail Making Test B: 66s (p50) (normal performances)

Verbal Fluency: phonemic category: 12 responses (norms 20.57 ± 5.99) (pathological performances)

Digit Span: forward 5; backward 4

The neuropsychological assessment showed preserved abilities in most cognitive domains such as episodic memory, but mild disturbances on executive functions (measures of working memory, retrieving information from memory) and visual memory. Otherwise on fluency tests, the production was also reduced.

33.5 Special Studies

Blood analysis: TSH: 1.294 mUI/L, T4: 18.2 pmol/L, T3: 4.39 pmol/L.

Brain MRI showed a mild cortical and subcortical atrophy without medial temporal and hippocampal atrophy.

The cerebrospinal fluid (CSF) analysis showed the following results:

Tau: 159 pg/L (N: 100–300 pg/L)

Abeta: 1015 pg/L (N: 500–1500 pg/L)

Ptau: 38 pg/L (N < 60 pg/L)

IATI score: 2.37

Protein 14-3-3: negative

Anti-central nervous system antibodies:

    Anti-rNMDA: negative

    Anti-LGI1: negative

    Anti-CASPR2: negative

Neuropil: atypical neuronal marking

The patient additionally performed an objective evaluation of the physical activity patterns using an ambulatory accelerometer (seven consecutive 24-h periods using a wrist-worn device on the non-dominant wrist) that did not reveal any changes in the rest-activity cycles.

33.6 Diagnosis

The patient was clinically diagnosed as having bipolar disorder without any associated neurodegenerative hypothesis.

33.7 Follow-Up

Considering the atypicity of the neuropil antibody results, Mrs. L, several months later, had a second CSF analysis that was not in favor of a dysimmune nor neurodegenerative disorder (Figure 33.1).

She also started an individual neuropsychological follow-up with implementation of cognitive (attention and concentration) training using MeMo (memory motivation training website). Indeed, despite a normal cognitive assessment, Mrs. L still expressed daily complaints and difficulties. It was thus important to be able to offer her adapted exercises, on a basis of ten 1-hour sessions, with a double goal: stimulate her cognitive abilities and improve her self-confidence by highlighting her success in the diverse exercises.

More specifically, on the cognitive level, the goals of the sessions were to improve her sustained and divided attention abilities, to stimulate her working memory, and to set up strategies allowing her to treat information faster and more efficiently.

Concerning long-term memory and learning capabilities, exercises such as learning and reminder of concrete visual scenarios, learning and reminder of 18, 20, 22, 24 concrete/abstract words with story creation, learning and reminder of heard stories with methodical selection of the information were used. Since Mrs. L did not show specific memory difficulties, she has been able to very quickly and autonomously set up learning strategies, which were efficient for her, easing encoding and recovery of information. Abilities of learning visual and verbal (seen or heard) information are functional. The

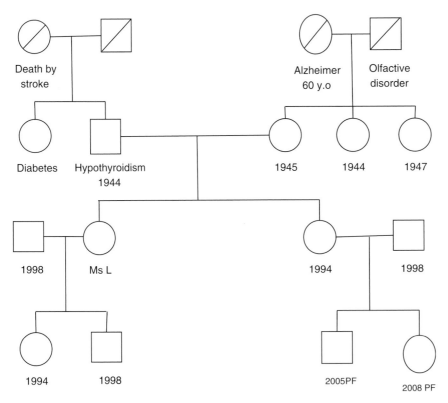

Figure 33.1 Mrs. L's genealogical tree. PF: periodic fever.

proposed exercises became more and more complex during the sessions and did not lead to objective difficulties.

Regarding attention and executive functions, the used exercises were, among others, crossing out in-line and in a heap concrete/abstract target(s), counting heard targets among distractors, managing various schedules. Along the sessions, Mrs. L improved her efficiency and speed in treating information, her concentration, sustained and selective attention capacities. Moreover, she is able to update information, and is not disturbed by interferences.

At last, concerning working memory, the used exercises were, for example, N-1 back tasks with numbers, pictures or words, multitask calculation, word completion from heard letters. Working memory abilities to handle multiple visual information are functional.

At the end of the individual care sessions, Mrs. L, still motivated and involved, had her improved performances on the memory as well as on the attention levels, whereas the proposed exercises were getting more and more complex. Without major difficulty, she has been reassured about her capabilities and did not need more sessions.

33.8 Discussion

Considering the patient's initial complaints (memory disturbances for recent facts) and her family history of early-onset AD, a cognitive assessment was legitimate despite her young age. BP elderly individuals have indeed an increased risk of dementia and usually perform worse on cognitive testings.[1]

At first consultation, Mrs. L had mild anxiety symptoms but was considered euthymic for the BP. The main cognitive disturbances reported among euthymic adults with bipolar disorder are executive disturbances, attention/working memory, speed/reaction time, verbal and visual memory.[2] Several mild cognitive disturbances observed for this BP euthymic patient are in agreement with the existing literature.

This young patient had the usual medical investigations (blood analysis and brain MRI). A lumbar puncture has been performed considering her executive and visual memory difficulties although she did not have verbal memory deficits. Her difficulties were not disabling but were seriously perturbating her daily life. A dosage of Alzheimer biomarkers was prescribed

and at the same time autoantibodies were analyzed to eliminate limbic encephalitis in face of cognitive troubles associated with psychiatric symptoms, even in the absence of an acute onset. The CSF analysis did not show any typical biological AD signature. In this line, one recent study, comparing CSF biomarkers between amnestic MCI individuals, AD individuals, and BP individuals with cognitive disturbances in late life, did not report a specific AD bio-signature among cognitively impaired BP individuals.[3]

In the present case, a cerebral PET imaging would have been useful in order to visualize metabolic patterns of neurodegenerative disease. So far, studies with FDG-PET have shown a pattern of corticolimbic metabolic dysregulation in BP, involving hypermetabolic rates in limbic structures and hypometabolism in frontal areas.[4] FDG-PET is routinely used to help to differentiate neurodegenerative diseases and is particularly interesting in investigating changes for early stages of the diseases.

More generally, cognitive changes in early-onset MCI (age < 65) remain underinvestigated compared to late-onset MCI. A study has shown that in a memory clinic, 12% of individuals with dementia were younger than 65. Among them, the most frequent diagnostic was MCI (18.7%) followed by AD and FTD.[5] It has been shown that individuals with younger age of onset have significantly longer time to first consultation and family awareness of the dementia diagnosis. The time to dementia diagnosis and to family awareness of dementia diagnosis was significantly longer when the participant presented with MCI. Perceived diagnostic delay may result in frustration and distress in patients with young onset dementia and their families.[6]

33.9 Take-Home Messages

1. Psychiatric disorders are frequently associated with cognitive impairments. The pattern of associated cognitive changes may resemble the cognitive impairments usually encountered among elderly individuals and should lead to further investigations for dementia syndrome despite existing psychiatric diagnoses (stabilized or not at the time of the consultation)
2. Young age at first presentation, independently of associated psychiatric disorders, should lead the clinician to propose more specific investigations such as CSF analysis or metabolic brain imaging.

References

1. Rise IV, Haro JM, Gjervan B. Clinical features, comorbidity, and cognitive impairment in elderly bipolar patients. *Neuropsychiatr Dis Treat.* 2016;12:1203–1213.

2. Cullen B, Ward J, Graham NA, et al. Prevalence and correlates of cognitive impairment in euthymic adults with bipolar disorder: a systematic review. *J Affect Disord.* 2016;205:165–181.

3. Forlenza OV, Aprahamian I, Radanovic M, et al. Cognitive impairment in late-life bipolar disorder is not associated with Alzheimer's disease pathological signature in the cerebrospinal fluid. *Bipolar Disord.* 2016;18(1): 63–70.

4. Scholl M, Damian A., Engler H, Fluorodeoxyglucose PET in neurology and psychiatry. *PET Clin.* 2014;9(4):371–390, v.

5. Croisile B, Tedesco A, Bernard E, et al. Diagnostic profile of young-onset dementia before 65 years. Experience of a French Memory Referral Center. *Rev Neurol (Paris).* 2012;168 (2):161–169.

6. Draper B, Cations M, White F, et al., Time to diagnosis in young-onset dementia and its determinants: the INSPIRED study. *Int J Geriatr Psychiatry.* 2016;31(11):1217–1224.

Concerns about the Future

Sarinporn Manitsirikul, Marlee Parsons, Monica Shin, Andrea L. Benedet, Tharick A. Pascoal, Mira Chamoun, Jean-Paul Soucy, Serge Gauthier, and Pedro Rosa-Neto

34.1 Clinical History

A 65-year-old accountant presented to the consultation to investigate whether her memory lapses are the first manifestations of Fahr's disease. She noticed, during the last few years, a progressive difficulty in accomplishing her tasks at work. She felt tired and described that it takes her more time to prepare her reports as compared to a few years ago. She needs to read her drafts several times in order to ensure her work is complete and accurate. She also described more dependence on her personal notes to remember her tasks such as lists for shopping. During meetings and conversations at work, she described difficulties recalling people's names. She has started to search for words during conversations. Although inconvenient, the impact of these difficulties on her work remains minimal, and she continues to take good care of her home affairs. Her husband denies that the patient is underperforming at home. She described no difficulties completing her domestic, financial, and personal obligations.

Ten years previously, she received the diagnosis of Fahr's disease following a brain CT conducted during a workup investigating headaches. The CT showed focal calcifications in caudate, thalami, cerebellar dentate nuclei, periventricular regions, and subcortical white matter, bilaterally. The ventricles and the rest of the brain parenchyma appeared normal. She was frightened with the possibility of becoming clinically symptomatic.

34.2 General History

The patient and her husband denied having recent sleep, cardiovascular, respiratory, or urinary problems. From the neuropsychiatric perspective, although the patient disclosed serious concerns about her future, there was no clinical history of disinhibition, reduced impulse control, substance-related disorders, stereotypical or ritualistic symptoms, hallucinations, or delusions.

34.3 Examination

Her neurological examination was normal. Her Montreal Cognitive Assessment (MoCA) score was 28/30 (impairment in naming and delayed recall). The Unified Parkinson's Disease Rating Scale (UPDRS) was unremarkable. From a cognitive perspective, she had normal executive functions, speed of processing, visual attention, visual memory, verbal memory, working memory, and social cognition.

Laboratory tests for calcium ion, phosphorus, magnesium, hepatic and renal function tests, protein electrophoresis, TSH, free T4, and parathyroid hormone were all normal. Microbiology tests for varicella zoster virus (VZV), Hepatitis B and C, and syphilis were negative.

Brain magnetic resonance imaging (MRI) showed hypodensity in T1W and hyperintensity in T2W region of the basal ganglia (bilaterally), and no acute ischemic changes were seen in DWI or ADC (Figure 34.1). [^{18}F]fluorodeoxyglucose (FDG) positron emission tomography (PET) scan showed decrease in cortical uptake in a non-systematic fashion, involving the right parietal lobe, left lower parietal lobe, bilateral precuneus (left worse than right), with sparing of the posterior cingulate giri. The right medial temporal lobe was also hypometabolic. The basal ganglia were markedly hypoactive. Thalamic uptake was normal. Cerebellar uptake was mildly decreased bilaterally (with right worse than left). Genetic analysis revealed a SLC20A2 mutation in c.1540delC (p.Leu514Trpfs*2).

34.4 Family History

The patient's mother died at the age of 83 years of massive gastrointestinal bleeding due to diverticulitis. Her father died at 55 years of intracerebral hemorrhage. The patient has one older sister, one younger brother, and two sons, all of whom are healthy. They refused to be assessed for basal ganglia calcification.

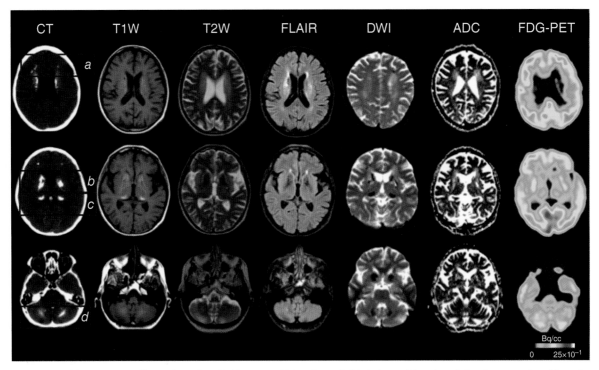

Figure 34.1 The images reveal hyperdense frontal white matter (a), basal ganglia (b), thalamus (c), and cerebellar dentate nucleus (d) on the CT scans. Correspondent basal ganglia hypointensity were observed in T1, T2W, FLAIR, DWI, and ADC images. FDG-PET images showed significant hypometabolism in the basal ganglia as well as temporal cortex.

34.5 Follow-Up

Five years later, she was clinically reassessed. She denied depression or abnormal movements. Her Mini-Mental State Examination (MMSE) score was 30/30, and her MoCA score was 30/30. The follow-up CT showed equivocal progression of white matter calcifications. The follow-up FDG-PET scan showed the same pattern of hypometabolism and decreased uptake at both frontal lobes (right more than left). Standardized scores on neuropsychological assessment remained normal; however, the scores for working memory were reduced as compared with her baseline assessment.

34.6 Diagnosis

The diagnosis of Idiopathic basal ganglia calcification (IBGC) seems appropriate given no evidence suggesting basal ganglia calcification in other family members. Although the genetic analysis was positive for a SLC20A2 mutation, the pathogenic correlation

to basal ganglia calcifications has not yet been established.

34.7 Discussion

Basal ganglia calcification (BGC) is an incidental finding in approximately 1% of head CT scans.[1–3] BGC may be caused secondary to hypoparathyroidism; pseudohypoparathyroidism; pseudopseudohypoparathyroidism; and other developmental, connective tissue, toxic, neoplastic, and infectious causes.[4] Idiopathic basal ganglia calcification (IBGC) has also been previously called primary familial brain calcification or Fahr's disease. IBGC is an infrequent disorder, clinically described as a progressive neurologic dysfunction starting in the fourth decade of life. However, IBGC phenotypes encompass a wide range of manifestations including cognitive impairment, psychiatric symptoms, and movement disorders in half of the cases. Headaches or seizures are also frequently reported. Importantly, a third of IBGC individuals remain asymptomatic.[5]

Given the high proportion of asymptomatic cases, the diagnosis of probable IBGC is primarily made on the basis of CT findings in the absence of underlying metabolic, infective, or other causes (secondary BGC). Interestingly, although the presence of calcifications is not enough to predict clinical presentations, there is a link between severity of the calcifications and clinical severity.[5] The genetic diagnosis permits definitive diagnosis of ambiguous cases.

Our case exemplifies the typical imaging presence of IBGC. The CT shows bilateral calcifications; MRI has high or low signal in T1 and low to isointense signal in T2 in the area of calcification. FDG–PET shows decreased uptake particularly in basal ganglia.[6] Importantly, the laboratory investigation in this patient was important to exclude secondary causes of BGC such as endocrinopathies (hypothyroidism, hypogonadotropism, and hypogonadism), systemic diseases (systemic scleroderma, systemic lupus erythematosus), infections (toxoplasmosis, neurocysticercosis, German measles, neurobrucellosis, HIV), primary or secondary calcified brain tumors, tuberous sclerosis, mitochondrial encephalopathy, myotonic muscle dystrophy, post-anoxia disorders, phacomatosis, Cockayne syndrome, idiopathic hemochromatosis, and heavy metal or carbon monoxide intoxication. A negative workup supports the diagnosis of probable IBGC.

Our patient has a new *SLC20A2* mutation in c.1540delC (p.Leu514Trpfs*2). This gene encodes the type III sodium-dependent phosphate transporter.[2] Alterations in this transporter may lead to calcium phosphate accumulation. The genetic underpinnings of IBGC show significant heterogeneity, and the complete description of contributing mutations is a topic of ongoing research. Mutations on the chromosome 5q32 (*PDGFRB* gene), chromosome 22q13.1 (*PDGFB* gene), and chromosome 1q25.3 (*XPR1* gene) have been associated with IBGC. As the variant in our patient has not been reported before, one can designate this as a variant of uncertain clinical significance (VOUS). As mentioned above, the familial form of IBGC, known as primary familial brain calcification (PFBC or Fahr's disease), is autosomal dominant and is phenotypically heterogeneous.[7–9]

34.8 Take-Home Messages

1. The diagnosis of probable IBGC is primarily made on the basis of CT findings in the absence of causative underlying metabolic, infective, or other causes (secondary BGC) and negative familial history.

2. Positive genetic testing diagnosis might confer the diagnosis of definitive IBGC, which includes multiple genes and a wide range of phenotypes.

3. As 30% of patients have negligible clinical manifestations, genetic counseling is crucial for patients' comprehension of risk of neurologic symptoms for themselves and their offspring.

References

1. Förstl H, Krumm B, Eden S, Kohlmeyer K. Neurological disorders in 166 patients with basal ganglia calcification: a statistical evaluation. *J Neurol.* 1992;239(1):36–38. doi:10.1007/BF00839209.

2. Harrington MG, Macpherson P, McIntosh WB, Allam BF, Bone I. The significance of the incidental finding of basal ganglia calcification on computed tomography. *J Neurol Neurosurg Psychiatry.* 1981;44(12):1168–1170. www.ncbi.nlm.nih.gov/pubmed/7334414. Accessed August 8, 2018.

3. Lauterbach EC, Cummings JL, Duffy J, et al. Neuropsychiatric correlates and treatment of lenticulostriatal diseases: a review of the literature and overview of research opportunities in Huntington's, Wilson's, and Fahr's diseases. A report of the ANPA Committee on Research. American Neuropsychiatric Association. *J Neuropsychiatr.* 1998; 10(3):249–66.

4. Manyam BV. What is and what is not "Fahr's disease". *Parkinsonism Relat Disord.* 2005;11(2):73–80. doi: 10.1016/j.parkreldis.2004.12.001.

5. Nicolas G, Pottier C, Charbonnier C, et al. Phenotypic spectrum of probable and genetically-confirmed idiopathic basal ganglia calcification. *Brain.* 2013;136(Pt 11):3395–3407. doi: 10.1093/brain/awt255.

6. Avrahami E, Cohn DF, Feibel M, Tadmor R. MRI demonstration and CT correlation of the brain in patients with idiopathic intracerebral calcification. *J Neurol.* 1994;241(6):381–384. doi: 10.1007/BF02033355.

7. Tadic V, Westenberger A, Domingo A, Alvarez-Fischer D, Klein C, Kasten M. Primary familial brain calcification with known gene mutations: a systematic review and challenges

of phenotypic characterization. *JAMA Neurol.* 2015;72 (4):460–467. doi: 10.1001/jamaneurol.2014.3889.

8. Hsu SC, Sears RL, Lemos RR, et al. Mutations in SLC20A2 are a major cause of familial idiopathic basal ganglia calcification. *Neurogenetics.* 2013;14(1):11–22. doi:10.1007/s10048-012-0349-2.

9. Wang C, Li Y, Shi L, et al. Mutations in SLC20A2 link familial idiopathic basal ganglia calcification with phosphate homeostasis. *Nat Genet.* 2012; 44(3):254–256. doi:10.1038/ng.1077.

Appendix: Diagnostic Criteria

1. Diagnostic Criteria for Creutzfeldt-Jakob Disease (CJD)[1]

1. Sporadic CJD

Possible

Rapidly progressive dementia; duration <2 years and at least two out of the following four clinical features:

1. Myoclonus
2. Visual or cerebellar signs
3. Pyramidal/extrapyramidal signs
4. Akinetic mutism

Probable (in the absence of an alternative diagnosis from routine investigation)

*Rapidly progressive dementia; duration <2 years and at least two out of the following four clinical features:

1. Myoclonus
2. Visual or cerebellar signs
3. Pyramidal/extrapyramidal signs
4. Akinetic mutism

*AND a positive result on at least one of the following laboratory tests:

1. A typical electroencephalogram (EEG) (generalized triphasic periodic complexes at approximately one per second), whatever the clinical duration of the disease, **and/or**
2. A positive 14-3-3 assay in cerebrospinal fluid (CSF)
3. MRI: high signal abnormalities in caudate nucleus and/or putamen on diffusion weighted imaging (DWI) or fluid attenuated inversion recovery (FLAIR)

Definite:

1. Neuropathological confirmation and/or presence of scrapie-associated fibrils
2. Confirmation of protease-resistant prion protein (PrP; immunocytochemistry or western blot); **and/or**
3. Presence of scrapie-associated fibrils

2. Iatrogenic CJD

Probable:
*Progressive cerebellar syndrome in a recipient of human cadaveric-derived pituitary hormone; or
*Sporadic CJD with a recognized exposure risk (e.g., antecedent neurosurgery with dura mater implantation)

Definite:
*Definite CJD with a recognized iatrogenic risk

3. Familial CJD

Probable
*Probable CJD plus confirmed or probable CJD in a first degree relative; and/or
*Neuropsychiatric disorder plus disease-specific prion protein gene (PRNP) mutation.

(cont.)

Definite:
*Definite CJD with a recognized pathogenic *PRNP* mutation; and
*Definite or probable transmissible spongiform encephalopathy (TSE) in a first-degree relative

Note. *For surveillance purposes, this definition includes Gerstmann-Sträussler-Scheinker (GSS) syndrome and fatal familial insomnia (FFI), and transmissible spongiform encephalopathy (TSE).*

4. Variant CJD

*Variant CJD (vCJD) cannot be diagnosed with certainty on clinical criteria alone; this requires neuropathological confirmation.
*The following combinations of signs, symptoms, and clinical investigations serve to define possible, probable, and definite vCJD:

(A)
*Progressive psychiatric disorder
*Clinical duration >6 months
*Routine investigations do not suggest an alternative diagnosis
*No history of potential iatrogenic exposure
*No evidence of a familial form of TSE

(B)
*Early psychiatric symptoms (depression, anxiety, apathy, withdrawal, delusions)
*Persistent painful sensory symptoms (pain and/or dysesthesia)
*Ataxia
*Chorea/dystonia or myoclonus
*Dementia

(C)
*A normal or an abnormal EEG, but not the diagnostic EEG changes often seen in classic CJD
*Bilateral symmetrical pulvinar high signal on MRI brain scan (relative to other deep gray-matter nuclei)
*Positive tonsil biopsy

vCJD Case Classification

Possible:
*A patient with the items under (A) above and at least four items under (B), EEG does not show the typical appearance of sporadic probable CJD
*A patient with the items under (A) and at least four items under (B)

Probable:
*A patient with the items under (A) and at least four items under (B)
*Bilateral pulvinar high signal on MRI brain scan
*EEG does not show the typical appearance of sporadic CJD although generalized periodic complexes may occasionally be seen at the later stages of the disease

OR:
*A patient with items under (A) and a positive tonsil biopsy.

Definite:
Neuropathological confirmation of vCJD
a. Numerous widespread kuru-type amyloid plaques surrounded by vacuoles in both the cerebellum and cerebrum - florid plaques
b. Spongiform change and extensive prion protein deposition shown by immunohistochemistry throughout the cerebellum and cerebrum

Note. *Tonsil biopsy not recommended routinely nor in cases with EEG appearances typical of sporadic CJD, but useful in suspect cases where clinical features are compatible with vCJD and MRI does not show high bilateral pulvinar signal.*

2. Diagnostic Criteria for Cortico-Basal Degeneration (CBD)[2]

Armstrong criteria: (A) proposed clinical phenotypes or syndromes; (B) proposed diagnostic criteria for CBD; (C) exclusion criteria for clinical research for both probable sporadic CBD and possible CBD

(A) Syndrome	Feature	
Probable CBD	Asymmetric presentation of two of (a) limb rigidity or akinesia, (b) limb dystonia, (c) limb myoclonus, plus two of (d) orobuccal or limb apraxia, (e) cortical sensory deficit, (f) alien limb phenomena (more than simple levitation)	
Possible CBD	(May be symmetric) One of (a) limb rigidity or akinesia, (b) limb dystonia, (c) limb myoclonus, plus one of (d) orobuccal or limb apraxia, (e) cortical sensory myoclonus, (f) alien limb phenomena (more than simple levitation)	
Frontal behavioral-spatial syndrome (FBS)	Two of (a) executive dysfunction, (b) behavioral or personality changes, (c) visuospatial deficits	
Non-fluent/agrammatic variant (NAV) of primary progressive aphasia	Effortful, agrammatic speech plus at least one of (a) impaired grammar/sentence comprehension with relatively preserved single-word comprehension or (b) groping, distorted speech production (apraxia of speech)	
Progressive supranuclear palsy syndrome (PSPS)	Three of (a) axial or symmetric limb rigidity or akinesia, (b) postural instability or falls, (c) urinary incontinence, (d) behavioral changes, (e) supranuclear vertical gaze palsy or decreased vertical saccade velocity	
(B)	Clinical research criteria for probable sporadic CBD	Clinical criteria for possible CBD
Presentation	Insidious onset and gradual progression	Insidious onset and gradual progression
Minimum duration of symptoms, years	1	1
Age at onset, years	≥ 50	No minimum
Family history (two or more relatives)	Exclusion	Permitted
Permitted phenotypes	(1) Probable CBD or (2) FBS or NAV plus at least one CBD feature (a–f).	(1) Possible CBD or (2) FBS or NAV or (3) PSPS plus at least one CBD feature (b–f).
Genetic mutation affecting tau (e.g., *MAPT*)	Exclusion	Permitted

(C) Exclusion criteria for clinical research for both probable sporadic CBD and possible CBD

Evidence of Lewy body disease, multiple system atrophy, Alzheimer's disease or amyotrophic lateral sclerosis, semantic or logopenic variant primary progressive aphasia, structural lesion suggestive of focal cause, granulin mutation or reduced plasma progranulin levels, TDP-43 or fused in sarcoma (FUS) mutations
Abbreviations: CBD, corticobasal degeneration; CBS, corticobasal syndrome; NAV, nonfluent/agrammatic variant.

3. Diagnostic Criteria for Progressive Supranuclear Palsy (PSP)[3]

Domain	Feature	Definition
*Ocular motor dysfunction		
O1	**Vertical supranuclear gaze palsy**	A clear limitation of the range of voluntary gaze in the vertical more than in the horizontal plane, affecting both up- and downgaze, more than expected for age, which is overcome by activation with the vestibulo-ocular reflex; at later stages, the vestibulo-ocular may be lost, or the maneuver prevented by nuchal rigidity.
O2	**Slow velocity of vertical saccades**	Decreased velocity (and amplitude) of vertical greater than horizontal saccadic eye movements; this may be established by quantitative measurements of saccades, such as infrared oculography, or by bedside testing; gaze should be assessed by command ("look at the flicking finger") rather than by pursuit ("follow my finger"), with the target >20° from the position of primary gaze; to be diagnostic, saccadic movements are slow enough for the examiner to see their movement (eye rotation), rather than just initial and final eye positions in normal subjects; a delay in saccade initiation is not considered slowing; findings are supported by slowed or absent fast components of vertical optokinetic nystagmus (i.e., only the slow following component may be retained).
O3	**Frequent macro square wave jerks or "eyelid opening apraxia"**	Macro square wave jerks are rapid involuntary saccadic intrusions during fixation, displacing the eye horizontally from the primary position, and returning it to the target after 200–300 ms; most square wave jerks are <1° in amplitude and rare in healthy controls, but up to 3–4° and more frequent (>10/min) in PSP. "Eyelid opening apraxia" is an inability to voluntarily initiate eyelid opening after a period of lid closure in the absence of involuntary forced eyelid closure (i.e., blepharospasm); the term is written in quotation marks because the inability to initiate eyelid opening is often attributed to activation of the pretarsal component of the orbicularis oculi (i.e., pretarsal blepharospasm) rather than failure to activate the levator palpebrae.
*Postural instability		
P1	**Repeated unprovoked falls within 3 years**	Spontaneous loss of balance while standing or history of more than one unprovoked fall, within 3 years after onset of PSP-related features.
P2	**Tendency to fall on the pull test within 3 years**	Tendency to fall on the pull test if not caught by examiner, within 3 years after onset of PSP-related features. The test examines the response to a quick, forceful pull on the shoulders with the examiner standing behind the patient and the patient standing erect with eyes open and feet comfortably apart and parallel.
P3	**More than two steps backward on the pull test within 3 years**	More than two steps backward, but unaided recovery, on the pull test, within 3 years after onset of PSP-related features.

(cont.)

Domain	Feature	Definition
*Akinesia		
A1	**Progressive gait freezing within 3 years**	Sudden and transient motor blocks or start hesitation are predominant within 3 years after onset of PSP-related symptoms, progressive and not responsive to levodopa; in the early disease course, akinesia may be present, but limb rigidity, tremor, and dementia are absent or mild.
A2	**Parkinsonism, akinetic-rigid, predominantly axial, and levodopa resistant**	Bradykinesia and rigidity with axial predominance, and levodopa resistance.
A3	**Parkinsonism with tremor and/or asymmetric and/or levodopa responsive**	Bradykinesia with rigidity and/or tremor, and/or asymmetric predominance of limbs, and/or levodopa responsiveness.
*Cognitive dysfunction		
C1	**Speech/language disorder**	Defined as at least one of the following features, which has to be persistent (rather than transient): 1. Nonfluent/agrammatic variant of primary loss of grammar and/or telegraphic speech or writing progressive aphasia (nfaPPA) or 2. Progressive apraxia of speech (AOS): Effortful, halting speech with inconsistent speech sound errors and distortions or slow syllabically segmented prosodic speech patterns with spared single-word comprehension, object knowledge, and word retrieval during sentence repetition.
C2	**Frontal cognitive/behavioral presentation**	Defined as at least three of the following features, which have to be persistent (rather than transient): 1. Apathy: Reduced level of interest, initiative, and spontaneous activity; clearly apparent to informant or patient. 2. Bradyphrenia: Slowed thinking; clearly apparent to informant or patient. 3. Dysexecutive syndrome: e.g., reverse digit span, Trails B or Stroop test, Luria sequence (at least 1.5 standard deviations below mean of age-and education-adjusted norms). 4. Reduced phonemic verbal fluency (e.g., "D, F, A, or S" words per minute; at least 1.5 standard deviations below mean of age- and education-adjusted norms). 5. Impulsivity, disinhibition, or perseveration (e.g., socially inappropriate behaviors, overstuffing the mouth when eating, motor recklessness, applause sign, palilalia, echolalia).
C3	**CBS**	Defined as at least one sign each from the following two groups (may be asymmetric or symmetric): 1. Cortical signs a. Orobuccal or limb apraxia b. Cortical sensory deficit c. Alien limb phenomena (more than simple levitation) 2. Movement disorder signs a. Limb rigidity b. Limb akinesia c. Limb myoclonus

(cont.)

Domain	Feature	Definition
*Clinical clues		
CC1	**Levodopa resistance**	Levodopa resistance is defined as improvement of the Movement Disorder Society-Sponsored Revision of the Unified Parkinson's Disease Rating Scale (MDS-UPDRS) motor scale by 30%; to fulfill this criterion patients should be assessed having been given at least 1,000 mg (if tolerated) at least 1 month OR once patients have received this treatment they could be formally assessed following a challenge dose of at least 200 mg.
CC2	**Hypokinetic, spastic dysarthria**	Slow, low volume and pitch, harsh voice.
CC3	**Dysphagia**	Otherwise unexplained difficulty in swallowing, severe enough to request dietary adaptations.
CC4	**Photophobia**	Intolerance to visual perception of light attributed to adaptative dysfunction.
*Imaging findings		
IF1	**Predominant midbrain atrophy or hypometabolism**	Atrophy or hypometabolism predominant in midbrain relative to pons, as demonstrated (e.g., by magnetic resonance imaging [MRI] or [^{18}F]fluorodeoxyglucose [FDG]- positron emission tomography [PET]).
IF2	**Postsynaptic striatal dopaminergic degeneration**	Postsynaptic striatal dopaminergic degeneration, as demonstrated (e.g., by [^{123}I] IBZM- single-photon emission computed tomography [SPECT] or [^{18}F]-DMFP-PET).

Degrees of diagnostic certainty, obtained by combinations of clinical features and clinical clues

Diagnostic Certainty	Definition	Combinations	Predominance Type	Abbreviation
Definite PSP	Gold standard defining the disease.	Neuropathological diagnosis	Any clinical presentation	def. PSP
Probable PSP	Highly specific, but not very sensitive for PSP.	(O1 or O2) (P1 or P2)	PSP with Richardson's syndrome	prob. PSP-RS
	Suitable for therapeutic and biological studies.	(O1 or O2) + A1	PSP with progressive gait freezing	prob. PSP-PGF
		(O1 or O2) (A2 or A3)	PSP with predominant parkinsonism	prob. PSP-P
		(O1 or O2) + C2	PSP with predominant frontal presentation	prob. PSP-F

(cont.)

Domain	Feature	Definition		
Possible PSP	Substantially more sensitive, but less specific for PSP.	O1	PSP with predominant ocular motor dysfunction	poss. PSP-OM
	Suitable for descriptive epidemiological studies and clinical care.	O2 + P3	PSP with Richardson's syndrome	poss. PSP-RS
		A1	PSP with progressive gait freezing	poss. PSP-PGF
		(O1 or O2) + C1	PSP with predominant speech/language disorder	poss. PSP-SL
		(O1 or O2) + C3	PSP with predominant CBD	poss. PSP-CBS
Suggestive of PSP	Suggestive of PSP, but not passing the threshold for possible or probable PSP.	O2 or O3	PSP with predominant ocular motor dysfunction	s.o. PSP-OM
		P1 or P2	PSP with predominant postural instability	s.o. PSP-PI
		O3 + (P2 or P3)	PSP with Richardson's syndrome	s.o. PSP-RS
		(A2 or A3) + (O3, P1, P2, C1, C2, CC1, CC2, CC3, or CC4)	PSP with predominant parkinsonism	s.o. PSP-P
		C1	PSP with predominant speech/language disorder	s.o. PSP-SL
		C2 + (O3 or P3)	PSP with predominant frontal presentation	s.o. PSP-F
		C3	PSP with predominant CBS	s.o. PSP-CBS

4. Diagnostic Criteria for Primary Progressive Aphasia (PPA)[4]

Diagnostic criteria for PPA

Inclusion: all criteria must be answered positively
1. Most prominent clinical feature is difficulty with language;
2. These deficits are the principal cause of impaired daily living activities;
3. Aphasia should be the most prominent deficit at symptom onset and for the initial phases of the disease.

Exclusion: all criteria must be answered negatively
1. Pattern of deficits is better accounted for by other non-degenerative nervous system or medical disorders;
2. Cognitive disturbance is a better accounted for by psychiatric diagnosis;
3. Prominent initial episodic memory loss, visual memory, and visuospatial impairments;
4. Prominent, initial behavioral disturbance.

Diagnostic features for the nonfluent/agrammatic variant PPA

I. Clinical diagnosis
A. One of the following core features must be present:
    1. Agrammatism in language production;
    2. Effortful, halting speech with inconsistent speech sound errors and distortions (apraxia of speech).
B. At least two of three of the following ancillary features must be present:
    1. Impaired comprehension of syntactically complex (noncanonical) sentences;
    2. Spared single-word comprehension;
    3. Spared object knowledge.

II. Imaging-supported nonfluent/agrammatic variant diagnosis
Both of the following criteria must be present:
1. Clinical diagnosis of nonfluent/agrammatic variant PPA;
2. Imaging must show one or more of the following results:
    a. Predominant left posterior fronto-insular atrophy on MRI or
    b. Predominant left posterior fronto-insular hypoperfusion or hypometabolism on SPECT or PET

III. Nonfluent/agrammatic variant PPA with definite pathology
Clinical diagnosis (criterion 1 below) and either criterion 2 or 3 must be present:
1. Clinical diagnosis of nonfluent/agrammatic variant PPA;
2. Histopathologic evidence of a specific neurodegenerative pathology (e.g., FTLD-tau, FTLD-TDP, AD, other);
3. Presence of a known pathogenic mutation.

Diagnostic criteria for the semantic variant PPA

I. Clinical diagnosis
A. Both of the following core features must be present:
    1. Impaired object naming;
    2. Impaired single-word comprehension
B. At least 3 of 4 of the following ancillary features must be present:
    1. Impaired object knowledge, particularly for low-frequency or low-familiarity items;
    2. Surface dyslexia or dysgraphia;
3. Spared repetition;
    4. Spared grammaticality and motor aspects of speech.

II. Imaging-supported semantic variant PPA diagnosis
Both of the following criteria must be present:
1. Clinical diagnosis of semantic variant PPA;
2. Imaging must show one or more of the following results:
    a. Predominant anterior temporal lobe atrophy;
    b. Predominant anterior temporal hypoperfusion or hypometabolism on SPECT or PET

(cont.)

III. Semantic variant PPA with definite pathology

Clinical diagnosis (criterion 1 below) and either criterion 2 or 3 must be present:

1. Clinical diagnosis of semantic variant PPA;
2. Histopathologic evidence of a specific neurodegenerative pathology (e.g., FTLD-tau, FTLD-TDP, AD, other);
3. Presence of a known pathogenic mutation.

Clinical diagnosis of logopenic variant PPA

I. Clinical diagnosis

A. Both of the following core features must be present:
1. Impaired single-word retrieval in spontaneous speech and naming;
2. Impaired repetition of phrases and sentences.

B. At least three of four of the following ancillary features must be present:
1. Phonological errors (phonemic paraphasias) in spontaneous speech or naming;
2. Spared single-word comprehension and object knowledge;
3. Spared motor speech;
4. Absence of frank agrammatism.

II. Imaging-supported logopenic variant diagnosis

Both criteria must be present:

1. Clinical diagnosis of logopenic variant PPA;
2. Imaging must show at least one of the following results:
   a. Predominant left posterior perisylvian or parietal atrophy on MRI
   b. Predominant left posterior perisylvian or parietal hypoperfusion or hypometabolism on SPECT or PET

III. Logopenic variant PPA with definite pathology

Clinical diagnosis (criterion 1 below) and either criterion 2 or 3 must be present:

1. Clinical diagnosis of logopenic variant PPA;
2. Histopathologic evidence of a specific neurodegenerative pathology (e.g., AD, FTLD-tau, FTLD-TDP, other);
3. Presence of a known pathogenic mutation.

5. Diagnostic Criteria for Lewy Body Dementia (LBD)[5]

Essential for a diagnosis of pretarsal component of the orbicularis oculi is dementia, defined as a progressive cognitive decline of sufficient magnitude to interfere with normal social or occupational functions, or with usual daily activities. Prominent or persistent memory impairment may not necessarily occur in the early stages but is usually evident with progression. Deficits on tests of attention, executive function, and visuo-perceptual ability may be especially prominent and occur early.

Core clinical features (The first three typically occur early and may persist throughout the course):

1. Fluctuating cognition with pronounced variations in attention and alertness.

2. Recurrent visual hallucinations that are typically well formed and detailed.

3. REM sleep behavior disorder, which may precede cognitive decline.

4. One or more spontaneous cardinal features of parkinsonism: these are bradykinesia (defined as slowness of movement and decrement in amplitude or speed), rest tremor, or rigidity.

Supportive clinical features

Severe sensitivity to antipsychotic agents; postural instability; repeated falls; syncope or other transient episodes of unresponsiveness; severe autonomic dysfunction (e.g., constipation, orthostatic hypotension, urinary incontinence); hypersomnia; hyposmia; hallucinations in other modalities; systematized delusions; apathy, anxiety, and depression.

Indicative biomarkers

Reduced dopamine transporter uptake in basal ganglia demonstrated by SPECT or PET.

Abnormal (low uptake) ^{123}iodine-MIBG myocardial scintigraphy.

Polysomnographic confirmation of REM sleep without atonia.

Supportive biomarkers

Relative preservation of medial temporal lobe structures on CT/MRI scan.

Generalized low uptake on SPECT/PET perfusion/metabolism scan with reduced occipital activity 6 the cingulate island sign on [^{18}F]FDG-PET imaging.

Prominent posterior slow-wave activity on EEG with periodic fluctuations in the pre-alpha/theta range.

Probable LBD can be diagnosed if

a. Two or more core clinical features of LBD are present, with or without the presence of indicative biomarkers, or

b. Only one core clinical feature is present, but with one or more indicative biomarkers.

Probable LBD should not be diagnosed on the basis of biomarkers alone.

Possible LBD can be diagnosed if

a. Only one core clinical feature of LBD is present, with no indicative biomarker evidence, or

b. One or more indicative biomarkers are present but there are no core clinical features.

LBD is less likely

a. In the presence of any other physical illness or brain disorder including cerebrovascular disease, sufficient to account in part or in total for the clinical picture, although these do not exclude a LBD diagnosis and may serve to indicate mixed or multiple pathologies contributing to the clinical presentation, or

b. If parkinsonian features are the only core clinical feature and appear for the first time at a stage of severe dementia.

6. Diagnostic Criteria for Posterior Cortical Atrophy (PCA)[6]

Core features of the PCA clinico-radiological syndrome (classification level 1)

Clinical features:

1. Insidious onset

2. Gradual progression

3. Prominent early disturbance of visual 6 other posterior cognitive functions

Cognitive features:

At least three of the following must be present as early or presenting features 6 evidence of their impact on activities of daily living:

1. Space perception deficit

2. Simultanagnosia

3. Object perception deficit

4. Constructional dyspraxia

5. Environmental agnosia

6. Oculomotor apraxia

7. Dressing apraxia

8. Optic ataxia

9. Alexia

10. Left/right disorientation

11. Acalculia

12. Limb apraxia (not limb-kinetic)

13. Apperceptive prosopagnosia

14. Agraphia

15. Homonymous visual field defect

16. Finger agnosia

All of the following must be evident:

Relatively spared anterograde memory function

Relatively spared speech and nonvisual language functions

Relatively spared executive functions

Relatively spared behavior and personality

Neuroimaging:

Predominant occipito-parietal or occipito-temporal atrophy/hypometabolism/hypoperfusion on MRI/[^{18}F]FDG-PET/SPECT.

Exclusion criteria:

Evidence of a brain tumor or other mass lesion sufficient to explain the symptoms

Evidence of significant vascular disease including focal stroke sufficient to explain the symptoms

Evidence of afferent visual cause (e.g., optic nerve, chiasm, or tract)

Evidence of other identifiable causes for cognitive impairment (e.g., renal failure).

Abbreviations: PCA, posterior cortical atrophy; MRI, magnetic resonance imaging; FDG-PET, ^{18}F-labeled fluorodeoxyglucose positron emission tomography; SPECT, single-photon emission computed tomography.

7. Diagnostic Criteria for Parkinson Disease (PD)[7]

The first essential criterion is parkinsonism, which is defined as bradykinesia, in combination with at least one of rest tremor or rigidity. Examination of all cardinal manifestations should be carried out as described in the MDS–Unified Parkinson Disease Rating Scale.

Once parkinsonism has been diagnosed

Diagnosis of Clinically Established PD requires

1. Absence of absolute exclusion criteria

2. At least two supportive criteria, and

3. No red flags

Diagnosis of Clinically Probable PD requires

1. Absence of absolute exclusion criteria

2. Presence of red flags counterbalanced by supportive criteria (No more than two red flags allowed)

   If one red flag is present, there must also be at least one supportive criterion.

   If two red flags, at least two supportive criteria are needed.

Supportive criteria

1. Clear and dramatic beneficial response to dopaminergic therapy. During initial treatment, patient returned to normal or near normal level of function. In the absence of clear documentation of initial response, a dramatic response can be classified as

(a) Marked improvement with dose increases or marked worsening with dose decreases. Mild changes do not qualify. Document this either objectively (>30% in UPDRS III with change in treatment) or subjectively (clearly documented history of marked changes from a reliable patient or caregiver).

(b) Unequivocal and marked on/off fluctuations, which must have at some point included predictable end-of-dose wearing off.

2. Presence of levodopa-induced dyskinesia

3. Rest tremor of a limb, documented on clinical examination (in the past or on current examination)

4. The presence of either olfactory loss or cardiac sympathetic denervation on MIBG scintigraphy.

Absolute exclusion criteria: The presence of any of these features rules out PD:

1. Unequivocal cerebellar abnormalities, such as cerebellar gait, limb ataxia, or cerebellar oculomotor abnormalities (e.g., sustained gaze evoked nystagmus, macro square wave jerks, hypermetric saccades)

2. Downward vertical supranuclear gaze palsy, or selective slowing of downward vertical saccades.

3. Diagnosis of probable behavioral variant frontotemporal dementia or primary progressive aphasia, defined according to consensus criteria within the first 5 years of disease.

4. Parkinsonian features restricted to the lower limbs for more than 3 years.

5. Treatment with a dopamine receptor blocker or a dopamine-depleting agent in a dose and time-course consistent with drug-induced parkinsonism. Absence of observable response to high-dose levodopa despite at least moderate severity of disease.

6. Unequivocal cortical sensory loss (i.e., graphesthesia, stereognosis with intact primary sensory modalities), clear limb ideomotor apraxia, or progressive aphasia.

7. Normal functional neuroimaging of the presynaptic dopaminergic system.

8. Documentation of an alternative condition known to produce parkinsonism and plausibly connected to the patient's symptoms, or, the expert evaluating physician, based on the full diagnostic assessment feels that an alternative syndrome is more likely than PD.

(cont.)

Red flags

1. Rapid progression of gait impairment requiring regular use of wheelchair within 5 years of onset.

2. A complete absence of progression of motor symptoms or signs over 5 or more unless stability is related to treatment.

3. Early bulbar dysfunction: severe dysphonia or dysarthria (speech unintelligible most of the time) or severe dysphagia (requiring soft food, NG tube, or gastrostomy feeding) within first 5 years.

4. Inspiratory respiratory dysfunction: either diurnal or nocturnal inspiratory stridor or frequent inspiratory sighs.

5. Severe autonomic failure in the first 5 years of disease. This can include:

(a) Orthostatic hypotension—orthostatic decrease of blood pressure within 3 min of standing by at least 30 mmHg systolic or 15 mmHg diastolic, in the absence of dehydration, medication, or other diseases that could plausibly explain autonomic dysfunction, or

(b) Severe urinary retention or urinary incontinence in the first 5 years of disease (excluding long-standing or small amount stress incontinence in women), that is not simply functional incontinence. In men, urinary retention must not be attributable to prostate disease, and must be associated with erectile dysfunction.

6. Recurrent (>1/year) falls because of impaired balance within 3 years of onset.

7. Disproportionate anterocollis (dystonic) or contractures of hand or feet within the first 10 years

8. Absence of any of the common non-motor features of disease despite 5 years of disease duration. These include sleep dysfunction (sleep-maintenance insomnia, excessive daytime somnolence, symptoms of REM sleep behavior disorder), autonomic dysfunction (constipation, daytime urinary urgency, symptomatic orthostasis), hyposmia, or psychiatric dysfunction (depression, anxiety, or hallucinations).

9. Otherwise-unexplained pyramidal tract signs, defined as pyramidal weakness or clear pathologic hyperreflexia (excluding mild reflex asymmetry and isolated extensor plantar response).

10. Bilateral symmetric parkinsonism. The patient or caregiver reports bilateral symptom onset with no side predominance, and no side predominance is observed on objective examination.

Criteria application:

1. Does the patient have parkinsonism, as defined by the MDS criteria?

   If "no," neither probable PD nor clinically established PD can be diagnosed. If "yes":

2. Are any absolute exclusion criteria present?

   If "yes," neither probable PD nor clinically established PD can be diagnosed. If "no":

3. Number of red flags present _____

4. Number of supportive criteria present _____

5. Are there at least 2 supportive criteria and no red flags?

   If "yes," patient meets criteria for clinically established PD. If "no":

6. Are there more than 2 red flags?

   If "yes," probable PD cannot be diagnosed. If "no":

7. Is the number of red flags equal to, or less than, the number of supportive criteria?

   If "yes," patient meets criteria for probable PD.

8. Diagnostic Criteria for Alzheimer Disease (AD)[8]

AD: (1) Probable AD dementia, (2) Possible AD dementia, (3) Probable or possible AD dementia with evidence of the AD pathophysiological process. The first two are intended for use in all clinical settings. The third is currently intended for research purposes.

1. Probable AD dementia: Core clinical criteria

A. Insidious onset. Symptoms have a gradual onset over months to years, not sudden over hours or days;

B. Clear-cut history of worsening of cognition by report or observation; and

C. The initial and most prominent cognitive deficits are evident on history and examination in one of the following categories:

   a. Amnestic presentation: It is the most common syndromic presentation of AD dementia. The deficits should include impairment in learning and recall on recently learned information. There should also be evidence of cognitive dysfunction in at least one other cognitive domain.

   b. Nonamnestic presentations:

*__Language presentation__: The most prominent deficits are in word-finding, but deficits in other cognitive domains should be present.

*__Visuospatial presentation__: The most prominent deficits are in spatial cognition, including object agnosia, impaired face recognition, simultagnosia, and alexia. Deficits in other cognitive domains should be present.

*__Executive dysfunction__: The most prominent deficits are impaired reasoning, judgment, and problem solving. Deficits in other cognitive domains should be present.

*__Note.__ The diagnosis of probable AD dementia **should not** be applied when there is evidence of (a) substantial concomitant cerebrovascular disease, (b) core features of Dementia with Lewy bodies other than dementia itself; or (c) prominent features of behavioral variant frontotemporal dementia; or (d) prominent features of semantic variant PPA or nonfluent/agrammatic variant PPA; or (e) evidence for another concurrent, active neurological disease, or a non-neurological medical comorbidity or use of medication that could have a substantial effect on cognition.*

1.1. **Probable AD dementia with increased level of certainty**
1.2.

1.1.1 Probable AD dementia with documented decline

In persons who meet the core clinical criteria for probable AD dementia, documented cognitive decline increases the certainty that the condition represents an active, evolving pathologic process, but it does not specifically increase the certainty that the process is that of AD pathophysiology.

Probable AD dementia with documented decline is defined as follows: evidence of progressive cognitive decline on subsequent evaluations based on information from informants and cognitive testing in the context of either formal neuropsychological evaluation or standardized mental status examinations.

1.1.2 Probable AD dementia in a carrier of a causative AD genetic mutation

In persons who meet the core clinical criteria for probable AD dementia, evidence of a causative genetic mutation (in APP, PSEN1, or PSEN2), increases the certainty that the condition is caused by AD pathology. The workgroup noted that carriage of the ε4 allele of the apolipoprotein E gene was not sufficiently specific to be considered in this category.

2. Possible AD dementia: Core clinical criteria

A diagnosis of possible AD dementia should be made in either of the circumstances mentioned in the following paragraphs.

Atypical course

Atypical course meets the core clinical criteria in terms of the nature of the cognitive deficits for AD dementia, but either has a sudden onset of cognitive impairment or demonstrates insufficient historical detail or objective cognitive documentation of progressive decline, or

(cont.)

Etiologically mixed presentation

Etiologically mixed presentation meets all core clinical criteria for AD dementia but has evidence of (a) concomitant cerebrovascular disease, defined by a history of stroke temporally related to the onset or worsening of cognitive impairment; or the presence of multiple or extensive infarcts or severe white matter hyperintensity burden; or (b) features of Dementia with Lewy Bodies other than the dementia itself; or (c) evidence for another neurological disease or a non-neurological medical comorbidity or medication use that could have a substantial effect on cognition.

Note: *A diagnosis of "possible AD" by the 1984 NINCDS-ADRDA criteria would not necessarily meet the current criteria for possible AD dementia. Such a patient would need to be reevaluated.*

3. Probable or possible AD dementia with evidence of the AD pathophysiological process

3.1 Probable AD dementia with evidence of the AD pathophysiological process

The major AD biomarkers that have been widely investigated at this time may be broken into two classes based on the biology which they measure:

A. Biomarkers of brain amyloid-beta (Aβ) protein deposition are low CSF Aβ42 and positive PET amyloid imaging.
B. The second category is that of biomarkers of downstream neuronal degeneration or injury.

The three major biomarkers in this category are elevated CSF tau, both total tau (t-tau), and phosphorylated tau (p-tau); decreased [^{18}F] FDG uptake on PET in temporo–parietal cortex; and disproportionate atrophy on structural magnetic resonance imaging in medial, basal, and lateral temporal lobe, and medial parietal cortex. T-tau and p-tau are treated equivalently in this study, although p-tau may have more specificity for AD than other dementing diseases.

In persons who meet the core clinical criteria for probable AD dementia biomarker evidence may increase the certainty that the basis of the clinical dementia diagnostic purposes at the present time. Syndrome is the AD pathophysiological process. However, we do not advocate the use of AD biomarker tests for routine.

3.2 Possible AD dementia with evidence of the AD pathophysiological process

This category is for persons who meet clinical criteria for a non-AD dementia but who have either biomarker evidence of AD pathophysiological process, or meet the neuropathological criteria for AD.

9. Diagnostic Criteria for Fronto-Temporal Dementia (FTD)[9]

International consensus criteria for behavioral variant FTD (bvFTD)

I. Neurodegenerative disease

The following symptom must be present to meet criteria for bvFTD:

A. Shows progressive deterioration of behavior and/or cognition by observation or history (as provided by a knowledgeable informant).

II. Possible bvFTD

Three of the following behavioral/cognitive symptoms (A–F) must be present to meet criteria. Ascertainment requires that symptoms be persistent or recurrent, rather than single or rare events.

A. Early* behavioral disinhibition [one of the following symptoms (A.1–A.3) must be present]:

A.1. Socially inappropriate behavior

A.2. Loss of manners or decorum

A.3. Impulsive, rash, or careless actions

B. Early apathy or inertia [one of the following symptoms (B.1–B.2) must be present]:

B.1. Apathy

B.2. Inertia

C. Early loss of sympathy or empathy [one of the following symptoms (C.1–C.2) must be present]:

C.1. Diminished response to other people's needs and feelings

C.2. Diminished social interest, interrelatedness, or personal warmth

D. Early perseverative, stereotyped, or compulsive/ritualistic behavior [one of the following symptoms (D.1–D.3) must be present]:

D.1. Simple repetitive movements

D.2. Complex, compulsive, or ritualistic behaviors

D.3. Stereotypy of speech

E. Hyperorality and dietary changes [one of the following symptoms (E.1–E.3) must be present]:

E.1. Altered food preferences

E.2. Binge eating, increased consumption of alcohol, or cigarettes

E.3. Oral exploration or consumption of inedible objects

F. Neuropsychological profile: executive/generation deficits with relative sparing of memory and visuospatial functions [all of the following symptoms (F.1–F.3) must be present]:

F.1. Deficits in executive tasks

F.2. Relative sparing of episodic memory

F.3. Relative sparing of visuospatial skills

III. Probable bvFTD

All of the following symptoms (A–C) must be present to meet criteria:

A. Meets criteria for possible bvFTD

B. Exhibits significant functional decline (by caregiver report or as evidenced by Clinical Dementia Rating Scale or Functional Activities Questionnaire scores)

(cont.)

   C. Imaging results consistent with bvFTD [one of the following (C.1–C.2) must be present]:

      C.1. Frontal and/or anterior temporal atrophy on MRI or CT

      C.2. Frontal and/or anterior temporal hypoperfusion or hypometabolism on PET or SPECT

IV. Behavioral variant FTD with definite FTLD Pathology

Criterion A and either criterion B or C must be present to meet criteria:

   A. Meets criteria for possible or probable bvFTD

   B. Histopathological evidence of FTLD on biopsy or at post-mortem

   C. Presence of a known pathogenic mutation

V. Exclusionary criteria for bvFTD

Criteria A and B must be answered negatively for any bvFTD diagnosis. Criterion C can be positive for possible bvFTD but must be negative for probable bvFTD.

   A. Pattern of deficits is better accounted for by other non-degenerative nervous system or medical disorders

   B. Behavioral disturbance is better accounted for by a psychiatric diagnosis

   C. Biomarkers strongly indicative of Alzheimer's disease or other neurodegenerative process

As a general guideline, 'early' refers to symptom presentation within the first 3 years. bvFTD = behavioral variant FTD.

10. Diagnostic Criteria for Frontal Variant of Alzheimer Disease (fvAD)[10]

Clinical features distinguishing frontal variant Alzheimer's disease (fvAD) from behavioral variant frontotemporal dementia (bvFTD):

	fvAD	bvFTD
Memory	Early memory complaints	Late memory complaints
Language	Phonemic and semantic paraphasias	Loss of socioemotional aspects of speech
Fluency	Semantic > phonemic fluency impairment	Phonemic > semantic fluency impairment
Behavioral	Compulsive or perseverative behaviors are uncommon	Collection or hoarding, and ritualistic and disinhibited behaviors (particularly involving food)
Personality Change	Agitation and irritability	Early apathy, disinhibition, loss of empathy
Thought Content	Delusions (theft, infidelity, and paranoia)	Mental rigidity
Body Habitus	Weight loss associated with depression	Weight gain associated with hyperphagia
Movement Disorder	Myoclonus (often mischaracterized as tremor), late parkinsonism	Early parkinsonism
Brain MRI pattern	Symmetric atrophy (temporal > frontal, posterior corpus callosum, and perisylvian)	Symmetric (~*MAPT* mutations) or asymmetric (~*GRN* mutations) frontotemporal atrophy
CSF findings	CSF p-tau/Aβ42 ratio (>0.21 ng/mL)	CSF progranulin levels (<60 ng/mL) – not validated in clinical practice
Biomarkers	APOE ε4 allele positive	No relation to APOE allele

11. Diagnostic Criteria for Vascular Dementia[11]

NINDS-AIREN

I. The criteria for the clinical diagnosis of probable vascular dementia include all of the following:

A. Dementia, defined by cognitive decline from a previously higher level of functioning and manifested by impairment of memory and of two or more cognitive domains (orientation, attention, language, visuospatial functions, executive functions, motor control, and praxis), preferably established by clinical examination and documented by neuropsychological testing; deficits should be severe enough to interfere with activities of daily living, not because of physical effects of stroke alone.

Exclusion criteria: cases with disturbance of consciousness, delirium, psychosis, severe aphasia, or major sensorimotor impairment precluding neuropsychological testing. Also excluded are systemic disorders or other brain diseases (such as Alzheimer's disease [AD]) that in and of themselves could account for deficits in memory and cognition.

B. Cerebrovascular disease, defined by the presence of focal signs on neurological examination, such as hemiparesis, lower facial weakness, Babinski sign, sensory deficit, hemianopia, and dysarthria consistent with stroke (with or without history of stroke), and evidence of relevant cerebrovascular disease (CVD) by brain imaging (computed tomography or magnetic resonance imaging [MRI]) including multiple large-vessel infarcts or a single strategically placed infarct (angular gyrus, thalamus, basal forebrain, or posterior cerebral artery or anterior cerebral artery territories), as well as multiple basal ganglia and white matter lacunes, or extensive periventricular white matter lesions, or combinations thereof.

C. A relationship between the above two disorders, manifested or inferred by the presence of one or more of the following:
   a. Onset of dementia within 3 months following a recognized stroke.
   b. Abrupt deterioration in cognitive functions.
   c. Fluctuating, stepwise progression of cognitive deficits.

II. Clinical features consistent with the diagnosis of probable vascular dementia include the following:

A. Early presence of gait disturbance (small-step gait or *marche à petits pas*, or magnetic, apraxic-ataxic, or parkinsonian gait).
B. History of unsteadiness and frequent, unprovoked falls.
C. Early urinary frequency, urgency, and other urinary symptoms not explained by urological disease.
D. Pseudobulbar palsy.
E. Personality and mood changes, abulia, depression, emotional incontinence, or other subcortical deficits including psychomotor retardation and abnormal executive function.

III. Features that make the diagnosis of vascular dementia uncertain or unlikely include the following:

A. Early onset of memory deficit and progressive worsening of memory deficit and progressive worsening of memory and other cognitive functions, such as language (transcortical sensory aphasia), motor skills (apraxia), and perception (agnosia) in the absence of corresponding focal lesions on brain imaging.
B. Absence of focal neurological signs, other than cognitive disturbance.
C. Absence of cerebrovascular lesions on brain CT or MRI.

IV. Clinical diagnosis of possible vascular dementia may be made in the presence of dementia (section I-A) with focal neurological signs in patients in whom brain imaging studies to confirm definite CVD are missing; or in the absence of clear temporal relationship between dementia and stroke; or in patients with subtle onset and variable course (plateau or improvement) of cognitive deficits and evidence of relevant CVD.

V. Criteria for diagnosis of definite vascular dementia are

A. Clinical criteria for probable vascular dementia.
B. Histopathological evidence of CVD obtained from biopsy or autopsy.
C. Absence of neurofibrillary tangles and neuritic plaques exceeding those expected for age.
D. Absence of other clinical or pathological disorder capable of producing dementia.

12. Diagnostic Criteria for Multiple System Atrophy (MSA)[12]

1. Criteria for the diagnosis of probable MSA

A sporadic, progressive, adult (>30 years) – onset disease characterized by
- Autonomic failure involving urinary incontinence (inability to control the release of urine from the bladder, with erectile dysfunction in males) or an orthostatic decrease of blood pressure, within 3 min of standing, by at least 30 mmHg systolic or 15 mmHg diastolic **and**
- Poor levodopa-responsive parkinsonism (bradykinesia with rigidity, tremor, or postural instability) **or**
- A cerebellar syndrome (gait ataxia with cerebellar dysarthria, limb ataxia, or cerebellar oculomotor dysfunction)

2. Criteria for possible MSA

A sporadic, progressive, adult (>30 years) – onset disease characterized by:
- Parkinsonism (bradykinesia with rigidity, tremor, or postural instability) **or**
- A cerebellar syndrome (gait ataxia with cerebellar dysarthria, limb ataxia, or cerebellar oculomotor dysfunction) **and**
- At least one feature suggesting autonomic dysfunction (otherwise unexplained urinary urgency, frequency or incomplete bladder emptying, erectile dysfunction in males, or significant orthostatic blood pressure decline that does not meet the level required in probable MSA) **and**
- At least one of the additional features (see point 2.1)

2.1 Additional features of possible MSA

Possible MSA-P or MSA-C
- Babinski sign with hyperreflexia
- Stridor

Possible MSA-P
- Rapidly progressive parkinsonism
- Poor response to levodopa
- Postural instability within 3 years of motor onset
- Gait ataxia, cerebellar dysarthria, limb ataxia, or cerebellar oculomotor dysfunction
- Dysphagia within 5 years of motor onset
- Atrophy on MRI of putamen, middle cerebellar peduncle, pons, or cerebellum
- Hypometabolism on FDG-PET in putamen, brainstem, or cerebellum

Possible MSA-C
- Parkinsonism (bradykinesia and rigidity)
- Atrophy on MRI of putamen, middle cerebellar peduncle, or pons
- Hypometabolism on FDG-PET in putamen
- Presynaptic nigrostriatal dopaminergic denervation on SPECT or PET

13. Diagnostic Criteria for Niemann-Pick Disease (NP)[13,14]

Niemann-Pick Disease Diagnostic criteria:

Type A and B also called Acid Sphingomyelinase Deficiency (ASMD)

Condition Description: Niemann-Pick disease types A and B are lysosomal storage disorders (LSD) caused by a defect in acid sphingomyelinase (ASM), resulting in accumulation of sphingomyelin. These are autosomal recessive disorders.

TYPE A (NP-A):

Consistent clinical findings and stereotypical course
- Massive organomegaly (hepatomegaly, splenomegaly)
- Eye findings: cherry red spots in the retina
- Lung disease and infections
- Cholesterol abnormalities
- Rapid progressive neurologic disease
- Failure to thrive
- Death by age of four

TYPE B (NP-B):

ASM deficient patients surviving early childhood more variability
- Eye findings in 34%
- Retinal findings were not a reliable predictor or the presence or severity of the neurologic findings
- Evidence of neurological involvements in 28%
- Progressive neurologic disease in less than 10%
- Interstitial lung disease and infections
- Most common disease are hypersplenism and dyslipidemia
- Progression lung disease occurs in most (interstitial lung disease)

Diagnostic Evaluation: Confirmatory sphingomyelinase enzyme assay. If low, the patient should have sphingomyelin phosphodiesterase 1 (*SMPD1*) gene analysis. Gene analysis may allow for separation of Type A from Type B.

TYPE C (NP-C):

NP-C disease is a neuro-degenerative disorder that can present at any age from newborn infants to adults. The fundamental problem in NPC is an accumulation of unesterified (free) cholesterol that is not available for cellular processes.

Clinical features indicating a possible diagnosis of NP-C:
- Fetal ascites or neonatal liver disease particularly when the latter is accompanied by prolonged jaundice and/or pulmonary infiltrates.
- Infantile hypotonia without evidence of progression for months to years followed by features outlined below:
  - Vertical supranuclear gaze palsy, progressive ataxia, dysartria, dystonia, and in some cases seizures, and gelastic cataplexy.
  - Onset of these symptoms on middle childhood, with progression over a course of years, in rare cases such presentations begin later in childhood or in adult life.
- Psychiatric presentation mimicking depression or schizophrenia, dementia starting during adolescence and adulthood.
- Enlargements particularly of the liver or spleen, particularly in early childhood.

Diagnostic Evaluation: Confirmed through biochemical and/or genetic testing

Type C is diagnosed using fibroblast cells from a skin biopsy. Cells from affected individuals show a reduced ability to transport cholesterol due to an inability to esterify it. Genetic testing is available from many laboratories for common mutations of the *NPC1* and *NPC2* genes.

References

1. Manix M, Kalakoti P, Henry M, et al. Creutzfeldt-Jakob disease: updated diagnostic criteria, treatment algorithm, and the utility of brain biopsy. *Neurosurg Focus.* 2015;39:E2.

2. Alexander SK, Rittman T, Xuereb JH, et al. Validation of the new consensus criteria for the diagnosis of corticobasal degeneration. *J Neurol Neurosurg Psychiatry.* 2014;85:925–929.

3. Hoglinger GU, Respondek G, Stamelou M, et al. Clinical diagnosis of progressive supranuclear palsy: the movement disorder society criteria. *Mov Disord.* 2017;32:853–864.

4. Henry ML, Gorno-Tempini ML. The logopenic variant of primary progressive aphasia. *Curr Opin Neurol.* 2010;23:633–637.

5. McKeith IG, Boeve BF, Dickson DW, et al. Diagnosis and management of dementia with Lewy bodies: fourth consensus report of the LBD Consortium. *Neurology.* 2017;89:88–100.

6. Crutch SJ, Schott JM, Rabinovici GD, et al. Consensus classification of posterior cortical atrophy. *Alzheimers Dement.* 2017;13:870–884.

7. Postuma RB, Berg D. The new diagnostic criteria for Parkinson's disease. *Int Rev Neurobiol.* 2017;132:55–78.

8. McKhann GM, Knopman DS, Chertkow H, et al. The diagnosis of dementia due to Alzheimer's disease: recommendations from the National Institute on Aging-Alzheimer's Association workgroups on diagnostic guidelines for Alzheimer's disease. *Alzheimers Dement.* 2011;7:263–269.

9. Rascovsky K, Hodges JR, Knopman D, et al. Sensitivity of revised diagnostic criteria for the behavioural variant of frontotemporal dementia. *Brain.* 2011;134:2456–2477.

10. Sawyer RP, Rodriguez-Porcel F, Hagen M, Shatz R, Espay AJ. Diagnosing the frontal variant of Alzheimer's disease: a clinician's yellow brick road. *J Clin Mov Disord.* 2017;4:2.

11. Erkinjuntti T. Clinical criteria for vascular dementia: the NINDS-AIREN criteria. *Dementia.* 1994;5:189–192.

12. Gilman S, Wenning G, Low PA, et al. Second consensus statement on the diagnosis of multiple system atrophy. *Neurology.* 2008;71:670–676.

13. Wraith JE, Imrie J. *Understanding Niemann-Pick Disease Type C and Its Potential Treatment.* Oxford: Blackwell Publ.; 2008.

14. Patterson MC, Clayton P, Gissen P, et al. Recommendations for the detection and diagnosis of Niemann-Pick disease type C An update. Neurology: Clinical Practice 2017:10.1212/CPJ. 0000000000000399.

Index